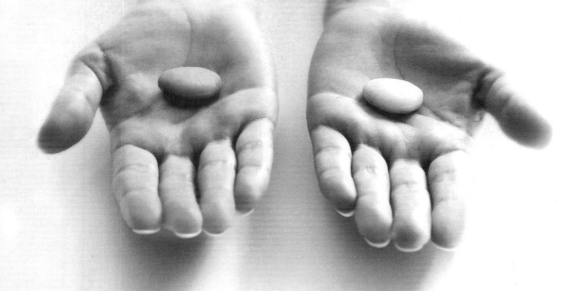

RISK AND CHOICE IN MATERNITY CARE

For Elsevier:

Commissioning Editor: Mary Seager; Mairi McCubbin
Development Editor: Rebecca Nelemans
Project Manager: Jane Dingwall
Design Direction: Judith Wright
Cover Design: Stewart Larking

RISK AND CHOICE IN MATERNITY CARE

An international perspective

Edited by

ANDREW SYMON

MA(Hons) PhD CTHE RGN RM

Senior Lecturer, School of Nursing and Midwifery, University of Dundee, UK

Foreword by

Professor Mavis Kirkham PhD RM RGN CertEd(Adult)

Professor of Midwifery, Sheffield Hallam University, UK

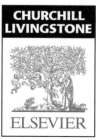

CHURCHILL LIVINGSTONE

ELSEVIER

Edinburgh London New York Oxford Philadelphia St Louis Sydney Toronto 2006

CHURCHILL
LIVINGSTONE
ELSEVIER

First published 2006

ISBN-10 0-443-10151-5
ISBN-13 978-0-443-10151-9

British Library Cataloguing in Publication Data
A catalogue record for this book is available from the British Library

Library of Congress Cataloging in Publication Data
A catalog record for this book is available from the Library of Congress

Printed in China by CTPS

Contents

Contributors

Pall Agustsson
Pall Agustsson is a Consultant in Obstetrics and Gynaecology at Ninewells Hospital, Dundee, Scotland. He has a special interest in obstetric ultrasound.

Janet Brooks CNM MPH
Janet Brooks has been a midwife for 17 years and is now working at the Monsey Family Health Center in Rockland County, New York. Janet is a NYS SAFE practitioner. She is a founding member and current President of the Board of Directors of Rockland Family Shelter in Rockland County, a full service agency for women and families affected by domestic violence.

Jennifer Cameron RN RM BAppSc (AdvNr/NrEd) MPH FRCNA FACM
Jennifer Cameron has held clinical, education and management positions in midwifery over the past 30 years. This experience was gained in public and private hospitals, academic institutions and hospital schools of nursing and midwifery. She has a strong interest in evidence-based practice and clinical risk management; in particular how individuals interpret and apply these concepts in practice. She is currently president of the NT branch of the Australian College of Midwives and is living in Darwin, practising midwifery.

Nadine Pilley Edwards PhD
Nadine Pilley Edwards is the Vice Chair of the Association for Improvements in the Maternity Services. She has been a birth activist and educator since 1976 and is currently a research associate in the School of Nursing and Midwifery at the University of Sheffield. She is the author of *Birthing Autonomy: Women's Experiences of Planning Home Births* and is now researching public participation through women's experiences of being on Maternity Service Liaison Committees.

David Ellwood MA DPhil FRANZCOG CMFM DDU
David Ellwood is Professor of Obstetrics and Gynaecology at The Australian National University Medical School and a subspecialist in maternal-fetal medicine. He is also the current President of the Perinatal Society of Australia and New Zealand. His clinical interests include the management of high-risk pregnancy and the use of ultrasound to monitor fetal wellbeing. He also has a long-standing interest in clinical risk management, particularly how it relates to the provision of maternity services in rural and remote areas. In 2001 he became the Chair of the Advanced Life Support in Obstetrics (ALSO) Advisory Board, which was responsible for introducing this course to Australia. The course has now been successfully delivered in many urban and

rural settings. He is a strong supporter of woman-centred, collaborative models of maternity care.

Brian Kennedy BA(Hons) MSc ACII
Brian Kennedy is a Director of Risk Management with Willis Limited, a global risk and insurance consultancy. He was jointly responsible for the creation and implementation of national risk management standards for the NHS in Scotland in 2001/02, and he has considerable experience of auditing healthcare risk management systems. His key interests are continuity planning, asset protection and safety, and within these areas he advises healthcare and corporate bodies alike.

Sinead McNally BA MSc MTD SRN SCM
Sinead McNally has been a midwife for almost 30 years, and a midwife teacher for 14 of those years. Her practice placement area during this time was Labour Suite. Weekly one-to-one teaching on the Labour Suite with students and mothers provided an opportunity to remain clinically credible and maintain 'hands on' skills. In 2000 Sinead was appointed as Clinical Risk Coordinator for Reproductive Health at the Simpson Centre for Reproductive Health (SCRH) in Edinburgh. She is an instructor for the Advanced Life Support in Obstetrics (ALSO) course, and teaches on local and international courses. At present she is studying for a Diploma in Risk Management.

Jo Murphy-Lawless BA MA PhD
Jo Murphy-Lawless, a sociologist, is currently at the School of Nursing and Midwifery, Trinity College Dublin. Involved in birth issues for over three decades in the UK and Ireland, she is author of *Reading Birth and Death: A History of Obstetric Thinking*.

Donna O'Boyle BSc MPhil LLB PGDip Forensic Medicine RN
Donna O'Boyle is a registered nurse and Director C3healthsolutions Ltd, Edinburgh, with a wide breadth of practice and professional qualifications in burns, intensive care, theatres and Accident & Emergency. The study of forensic medicine and then law to degree and master's levels stimulated her interest in medico-legal issues. As former Head of Clinical Risk at a large London teaching trust, and latterly as CNORIS (Clinical Negligence and Other Risks Indemnity Scheme) clinical assessor for the NHS in Scotland, Donna has a wide knowledge of the impact of adverse incidents and litigation on practitioners and clients alike. A great believer in the potential of properly informed staff to contribute to the patient safety agenda, Donna facilitates risk management and healthcare governance support to staff across healthcare in the UK, delivering help in understanding the legal and practical implications of consent, learning from adverse events and other topics supporting safer and improved quality of care.

Marie O'Connor
Marie O'Connor is a sociologist, researcher and health activist who has written extensively on birth and maternity care. Her interests include women's health, gender, power and public policy. *Birth Tides* (Pandora, London, 1995), her study of home birth commissioned by the Irish Department of Health, exposed, for the first time in its country of origin, the harsh reality of women's experiences of active management. She is currently completing a book on the crisis in Irish healthcare and has been active in health politics for 25 years. Her work has been translated into a number of European languages.

Mike Rich
Mike Rich has been the Chief Executive of the charity Action on Pre-eclampsia for the past 4 years. His background is not in medicine but in the voluntary sector where he has been, among other things, the Head of Public Affairs at a major children's charity and the Head of Development at an adoption and fostering charity.

Lesley Anne Smith MB ChB
Lesley Anne Smith is the Head of Clinical
Governance and Risk Management at NHS
Highland. She gained her MB ChB from
Aberdeen University in 1983 and worked as
a junior doctor for several years before
training as a chartered accountant. She has
worked in the clinical governance field for
5 years and has been a member of the
national Healthcare Governance Standards
Steering Group established by NHS Quality
Improvement Scotland to develop clinical
governance and risk management standards.
She is also a member of the national working
group established to produce the report
*Managing the Risks of Healthcare Associated
Infection* for NHS Scotland.

Andrew Symon MA(Hons) PhD CTHE, RGN RM
Andrew Symon is Senior Lecturer in
the School of Nursing and Midwifery at the
University of Dundee, and is the

postgraduate academic facilitator for the
MSc Advanced Practice (Midwifery). His
interest in risk and choice stems from
his PhD (University of Edinburgh, 1997),
which examined the incidence and effects of
perinatal litigation. He has published two
books based on this research, and co-edited a
third on clinical risk management. Current
research interests include the assessment of
quality of life, and the effects of interior
design on women and staff in maternity
units.

Denis Walsh, MA PhD PGDipEd RM DPSM
Denis Walsh is an Independent Midwifery
Consultant and runs the Evidence Course for
Midwives internationally. He is also a Senior
Lecturer in Midwifery at the Midwifery
Research Centre at the University of Central
Lancashire, Preston. His research interests
are normal birth, birth centres and
midwifery-led models of care.

Foreword

In modern maternity care rhetoric, risk is usually defined by professionals and imparted by them to service users. The consumers of services then make choices, usually of compliance with the professionally proposed course of action, in the light of the risks outlined. This book enables us to see risk and choice more analytically.

Service users in Scotland, Ireland and Australia bring different values and concepts of safety and differing health professions offer a range of viewpoints. Research from many disciplines is used by chapter authors. The wide range of contributions offers us glimpses of other definitions of safety, beside those contained within the parameters of a profession. Equally, we are afforded glimpses from viewpoints where values differ.

The various analyses of risk and choice, and how these concepts are linked, give us insight into the values and priorities which underpin how risk is conceptualised, presented and managed. Similarly we can draw insight into the construction of choice. The essentially political nature of risk discourses is thus demonstrated in the variety of views offered.

This edited collection is contained between a clear introduction on the risk–choice paradox and a thoughtful concluding chapter on knowledge and control. As such, it is well constructed and challenging.

This book makes an important contribution to the debate on risk and choice in maternity care. Reading the range of approaches to risk here should open up possibilities for the reader to explore risk, rather than accept it as defined. Such exploration can be enabling, for parents and for professionals. Many choices made in assessing risk lie implicit, but can be identified. This book equips us to do that.

Sheffield, 2006   Mavis Kirkham

Preface

Risk is one of those aspects of modern life that almost needs no introduction. The term is used freely and widely, but this is perhaps one of its drawbacks. Likewise, choice is a part of our post-modern world, when most of those in developed countries live in a world of choices and opportunities. However, yet again the initial impression – that we know what choice is – may be misleading. What do these features actually mean in terms of maternity care?

Risk and Choice in Maternity Care is not a polemic on the rights and wrongs of the debate over whether choice can truly be offered, nor a critique of Beck's *Risk Society*. What it does is to set the maternity care scene by describing how different players tackle these issues. Taking an international perspective, it sheds light on how midwives, pregnant women, obstetricians and risk managers approach these subjects. A truly comprehensive book would have to cover an enormous range of countries and viewpoints *Risk and Choice in Maternity Care* sets out to open up the debate from a range of perspectives in a number of countries.

The book presents viewpoints from a wide range of professional and informed lay positions in the UK, Ireland, the USA and Australia. It not only answers some people's questions, but it also poses new questions about this complex subject.

Dundee, 2006

Andrew Symon

Acknowledgements

When naming those who helped in the production of a book there is a terrible risk of offending people who aren't included.

Many people helped, both in Dundee and at Elsevier: you know who you are. Thank you.

Chapter 1

The Risk–Choice Paradox

Andrew Symon

INTRODUCTION

Risk and choice are two contemporary themes that command a great deal of attention. While it can be argued that Western societies have become risk-conscious to an extraordinary extent, and that this has led to a culture of fear which constrains freedom of activity, at the same time choice is one of the great mantras of the modern age. There is a paradox here: while it is claimed that people are increasingly aware of risks and dangers, and consequently fearful of adverse outcomes, there is at the same time at least an apparent demand for freedom of choice.

Reports of risk awareness (or indeed risk aversion) cover many aspects of contemporary life. Some media stories delight in the coverage of apparently absurd accounts of organisations being unwilling to accept even minuscule risks for fear of poor outcomes and even litigation. At the same time advertising offers the apparent possibility of a wide range of consumer choices, whether this relates to merchandise or lifestyle, and there is a corresponding drive towards making such choices. Contemporary politics seems to thrive on the depiction of fear: fear of crime or concerns over national security are a staple part of political debate, yet even on these subjects the various political parties often strive to offer alternatives – in other words, a choice.

Concerns and periodic panics over the safety of food or environmental pollution reflect widespread fears about how large populations may be put at risk. Apprehension over the cumulative impact of many individual examples of untoward outcomes has led to a rapid growth of risk management within the health services in the past decade in an attempt to limit the emotional, clinical and legal-financial consequences of such events. Despite the apparently constraining effects of these phenomena, at the same time government policy in the UK has been stressing the importance of choice for healthcare 'consumers' (DH 2004).

The situation is perhaps most acute within maternity care, where expectations are high and the fear of loss most accentuated. While on the one hand the fall in maternal and perinatal mortality rates over the past 50 years in Western countries ought to have instilled a greater confidence in childbirth, this is offset by reports of potentially dangerous healthcare and a terror of poor outcomes (Johnson & Slade 2002). While these reports may be unrepresentative of the big picture, their impact on public trust in healthcare providers can be immense. If the effect of such stories is to make people fearful of poor outcomes, and consequently averse to taking what are seen as unacceptable risks, where does that leave the exercise of choice?

This chapter, drawing principally on the experience in Britain, will attempt to unravel some of these issues, and introduce the reader to some of the themes explored throughout the book. It will question whether risk and choice in maternity care, being related to much wider concerns within society, are necessarily as oppositional as they are sometimes portrayed to be. It is a complex and evolving subject, and healthcare users and providers must try to make sense of an intricate mosaic of facts, opinions and reportage.

THE GREAT RISK DEBATE

The management of risk has become a growth industry. The origins of this phenomenon are laudable enough – there is a desire to protect what is precious and valued. Health and safety rules are there to protect employees and others from certain risks. However, there seems to be a variance of opinion about what 'risk' actually means. A scientific categorisation might include something along the lines of the statistical likelihood of a given hazard occurring. (It should be noted that 'risk' usually has a negative connotation; when people talk about a positive outcome, they say there is an X *chance* of this happening.) In spite of the theoretical objectivity of such a position, how this translates into public perception is not always straightforward. There are claims that people routinely exaggerate some low risks which have a high potential impact (such as plane crashes), while depreciating higher risks that are perceived to have a lower impact (such as multiple car journeys). The upshot is that some people are deterred from flying even though, statistically speaking, they are safer travelling by plane than by car (Bellaby 2001).

Healthcare is certainly not an isolated field in this regard. As a concept, 'risk' applies to almost any subject one cares to mention – food and travel are good examples. Paradoxically, the desire to minimise risk and to try to ensure some degree of safety has led to a backlash to what some may call the 'nanny state', whereby some people actively seek out risky situations – 'extreme sports' such as sky-diving being a case in point. Adams (1995) posits the theory that we all have a 'risk thermostat', and that we adjust our behaviour in order to maintain what we deem to be an acceptable level of risk. This brings into question how risk is perceived and communicated.

Relative risks are one way of trying to explain the likelihood of a given occurrence. Smith (2002) presents a 'risk ladder', which explains the relative likelihood of different occurrences. For example, there is less than a 1 in 100 000 risk of getting a spinal haematoma following an epidural, while the risk of dying in a road traffic accident is around 1 in 10 000. Statistically, one is about 10 times more likely than the other, but this doesn't mean that someone would be less apprehensive about having an epidural than of getting in a car. We accept and deal with certain risks, while others that are less likely and even less serious in terms of outcome, are judged unacceptable.

The desire to quantify risks has led to the concept of risk assessment, whereby locations or situations are appraised with a view to judging their safety. This has led to some unintentionally humorous examples. A recent media report noted that warnings about confidence tricksters could not be printed on paper napkins delivered to elderly people along with their cooked meals (part of the 'meals-on-wheels' service offered by some local councils). This resulted from a risk assessment exercise which felt that the napkins were a choking hazard. A representative of the local pensioners' forum commented 'To risk-assess a napkin is utterly ridiculous and an unnecessary cost to the taxpayer' (Wainwright 2005). Such examples aside, few would disagree that the process of trying to minimise harmful occurrences is a good thing. The Health and Safety Executive (HSE), the body responsible for health and safety issues arising from work activity in Britain, notes that:

> A risk assessment is nothing more than a careful examination of what, in your work, could cause harm to people, so that you can weigh up whether you have taken enough precautions or should do more to prevent harm. The aim is to make sure that no one gets hurt or becomes ill.
>
> (HSE 1999: 2)

This is fairly uncontroversial. Most people take certain steps to ensure their own safety in their everyday lives, and the HSE approach is no more than codifying for work premises what is felt to be good and reasonable practice in this regard. While the most obvious benefits may be seen in 'heavy industries' (e.g. large-scale manufacturing plants), with safety mechanisms added to machines, the principles apply to all workplaces, including offices and hospitals. There is still the element of choice: a worker may decide not to use the advised protective equipment, for example.

RISK IN HEALTHCARE

Risk considerations have acquired considerable resonance within healthcare over the past decade or so, and maternity care in particular has been the focus of much debate about direction, process and outcomes. In the wider health field there has been an explosion of interest in risk: journals such as *Clinical Risk*, the *Health-Care Risk Report* and *Health, Risk and Society* offer insights into the nature and implications of risk. Books on the subject include *Medicine, Health and Risk* (Gabe 1995a) and *Risk Management in Health Care Institutions* (Kavaler & Spiegel 2003). More specific references to maternity care include *Risk Management and Litigation in Obstetrics and Gynaecology* (Clements 2001), *Clinical Risk Management in Midwifery* (Wilson & Symon 2002), and *Litigation: a risk management guide for midwives* (RCM 2005). Formalised risk management systems have been in place in the National Health Service for several years now, prompted partly by the prospect of a litigation/compensation crisis (cf. Symon 2001). The National Health Service Litigation Authority (NHSLA), set up in 1995, spawned the Clinical Negligence Scheme for Trusts (CNST) in England, and risk management standards, based on the Australian-New Zealand standards (AS/NZS 2004) have been implemented; this is considered fully by Kennedy in Chapter 2. (The Scottish and Welsh equivalents, respectively, are CNORIS (Clinical Negligence and Other Risks Indemnity Scheme), and the Welsh Risk Pool.) The consciously medico-legal approach to risk management is exemplified by the Royal College of Midwives' statement that 'The current risk approach to maternity care has created a climate in which the fear of litigation has thrived' (RCM 2003: 1). The National Patient Safety Agency (NPSA) was set up in England in 2001 to coordinate all aspects of safety in healthcare through the collection and analysis of relevant information and the dissemination of advice on how best to maximise safety. It can be seen that there is no shortage of information and opinion on the subject of risk in healthcare, with maternity care playing a prominent role.

Despite this apparent knowledge about what risk is and the way in which it might be managed, how health risks are perceived is a subject of great debate. Media stories about dangerous substances in food produce periodic panics despite food recalls and/or official information that the risk is minuscule (Doyle 2004, BBC 2005). Harrabin et al (2003) note that the media do not view or report risk in the same 'intellectual' way as doctors, government officials and scientists. They report the view that people have difficulty in interpreting statistics that do not have an emotional charge. In this way the severity of a possible outcome becomes more important than its probability. It is not hard to see how this skewed translation of data can produce unintended effects in healthcare discussions. In this vein Gabe (1995b) notes how a few reported cases about necrotising fasciitis became a media horror story about 'killer bugs' that threatened public safety. More recent media stories about a possible avian flu pandemic have again shown how difficult it can be to evaluate risk.

News stories about other potential health risks, such as the possibility that the combined MMR (measles, mumps and rubella) vaccine may predispose to or cause autism in some children, can also cause concern on a general level. Bellaby (2003: 726) notes that parental unease about the vaccine affected health professionals, but says that it is a mistake to conclude that the media simply misled the public. Earlier government denials about other possible dangers (e.g. eating beef following the 'mad cow disease' scares) were treated with scepticism by many, and this led some to be cynical about official claims concerning safety.

The media have been criticised for presenting an imbalanced view of different risks. Harrabin et al (2003: 14), in what they concede is a crude measure of mortality risk associated with a particular condition or behaviour, note that '8,571 people died of smoking for each smoking story on the BBC news. It took only 0.33 deaths from vCJD [variant Creutzfeldt–Jakob disease] to merit a story.' While there are undoubtedly many media stories that give an unrepresentative picture of different risks, this is not a universal feature of media reporting. The Social Issues Research Centre (SIRC), based in Oxford, England, claims to publish a regular 'Naming and Praising' (as opposed to 'Naming and Shaming') column, highlighting examples of scare-proof reporting. They say that journalists should be praised for refusing to exaggerate risks for the sake of an eye-catching headline, and note that it is from 'the interpretation of the findings and in generalisations made from limited data that misrepresentations are most likely to arise' (SIRC 2000).

Taking this away from general portrayals of possible health risks onto the individual level, there can be difficulties in trying to communicate risks or certain outcomes, not least because some practitioners are themselves not aware of the true extent of the risk (Woloshynowych & Adams 1999). Trying to communicate risk levels when large numbers are involved can also be problematic. One solution is to offer pictograms such as the Paling palettes (Paling 1997) or graphic 'risk language proposals' (Edwards et al 2002). However, even here there may be difficulties in applying the concept of a certain level of risk to oneself: 'What I wanted to know . . . was "Will it happen to me?". . . To a large extent, the interpretation of the statistics comes down to whether you are an optimist or a pessimist' (Quilliam 1999: 282).

Risk in the context of maternity care is an often contentious subject, with risk being used as a label that denotes suitability for particular models of care. This is especially relevant given changing patterns of service delivery within Britain. Recent years have seen a shift to a concentration of large obstetric units for women deemed 'high' or 'medium' risk, and developments within midwife-led care for women deemed 'low risk'. Not all midwives, it seems, quickly adapt to the 'low risk' approach to maternity care currently being advocated (NHS MA 2004). Within Scotland it is acknowledged that this shift in focus is away from one of 'need' and towards one of 'risk' (EGAMS 2002). The different interpretations brought to the understanding of the word 'risk' in this context underlie the sometimes vexatious debates about choice and the appropriateness of different care packages. Despite the low specificity of tools designed to predict risk, healthcare practitioners, socialised into an epidemiological understanding of morbidity, may view the application of a 'risk label' as a means of trying to ensure a positive clinical outcome. Pregnant women's understanding of 'risk' – without wanting to generalise too much – is said to be more contextual, being embedded in their own particular lives (Stahl & Hundley 2003), with a correspondingly lower perception of the likelihood of an adverse outcome. Edwards & Murphy-Lawless consider this in detail in Chapter 4. What this leaves women by way of control over choice of place of birth or type of care, is the subject of debate. It should also be borne in mind that there is a public health dimension to managing risk which may not sit easily within a purely individualist approach.

CHOICE IN HEALTHCARE

CHOICES, CHOICES

As noted above, choice is one of the mantras of the modern age. A central feature of advanced capitalist societies is that products and markets are consumer-driven: only those products and services that are feasible and desirable will remain viable. This assumes that people make rational choices, and indeed that they are in a position to do so. There are economic critiques of such a view – those marginalised in economic terms often do not have the luxury of making choices. There is also criticism that choice is often chimera: there is the initial perception of choice, before the realisation that this is either limited or non-existent, reflecting the dictum attributed to Henry Ford: 'You can have any colour you want, as long as it's black.'

Developed industrialised societies exist on the understanding that economic growth is both necessary and desirable. The 'consumer society' requires constant adaptation in goods and services, and so new products are forever appearing, offering those with sufficient wherewithal the chance to purchase them. The notion of choice implies a certain level of information and understanding: people choose products or services because they understand that they

want or need them, and that they are able to distinguish those products from others that either appear similar or offer alternatives. How people acquire such understanding, in general terms as well as within healthcare, is complex. Information may be available in the form of product news or advertising, but only the most naïve will take all of this on trust. Personal recommendations are highly valued as individualised forms of evidence. Thornton (2003: 694) acknowledges that practitioners must develop partnerships with users 'to examine social factors that go beyond the cognitive to the behavioural, including the social context in which meanings are shaped.'

There are different models of healthcare within the developed world. It can be argued that in a fee-for-service model, choices can be made as in any other area of economic activity: if the market will sustain the option, then it should be made available. This is particularly relevant when considering certain choices made in maternity care: if a woman is willing to pay, should she be free to choose a caesarean section for which there is no obvious clinical indication? This illustrates the developing complexity when choice is introduced into healthcare discussions. Quite apart from financial considerations, there may be ethical issues involved in certain courses of action. Within Britain the rhetoric of 'choice' became more pronounced with the introduction of strategic reforms in the 1980s and 1990s. Consciously political in tone, these changes were intended to make the health service less centralist and more responsive to what can be called market-oriented demands. This debate quickly centres on what is said to be 'informed choice', and the concept on which this is premised, 'evidence-based' care.

It is possible to be cynical about the rhetoric of choice (cf. Anderson 2004). Informed decision-making requires a level of knowledge and understanding. Many women will come to antenatal visits with a great deal of both, but with a reduced routine antenatal visit schedule, and pressure of time during antenatal clinics, there may be little time for practitioners to provide information, never mind discuss matters with the woman. Godolphin (2003: 692), referring to formative medical training, notes that most of this takes place in acute care situations, when practitioners 'are taught to be responsible in settings where choices are few and patients' autonomy is limited'. It can be argued that a similar position has existed in midwifery, although a greater focus on continuity of carer and in involving women ought, in theory, to have offset this. Also compensating for this is the trend towards delivering less pregnancy care in hospitals and more in the community, where the setting is more relaxed and there is usually slightly less pressure of time.

Hewson (2004: 32) notes that the social context in which these discussions take place has changed significantly: 'women no longer expect a highly paternalistic model of care, and are more likely to question, or even to reject, professional advice.' She goes on to note that while this may hold true in Britain, it is not universally the case. She cites Ireland as an example of where women are expected to accept a medically-determined pattern of care. This is considered later in this book by O'Connor. If, in some countries at least, women expect to have a say in the care package that is decided on, how do they reach their decisions about care, and how are these preferences made known?

EVIDENCE

The term 'evidence' is used widely to denote a superior standard. 'Evidence' is held to be proof (as in a court of law), but there are many different versions of evidence. Healthcare practitioners, as noted above, may be socialised into an acceptance of the epidemiological model of healthcare planning. This statistically-driven model produces categories based on aggregated data, and these can be used to inform care management plans. For instance, data about the relative risks associated with vaginal birth after more than one caesarean section can be used to advise a pregnant woman about mode of delivery (cf. AIMS 2004). On one level, this type of evidence is highly persuasive: a

professionally-controlled agenda sets great store by such data, arguing on utilitarian grounds that this approach ensures the greatest likelihood of a good clinical outcome on a population level. On the other hand, a woman may believe that, previous scars on her uterus notwithstanding, she has the ability to achieve a normal vaginal birth, and so may disregard what some health professionals will see as straightforward commonsense advice. Perhaps somewhere in the middle there may be practitioners who want to promote the woman's autonomy with regard to decision-making, but who are mindful that they work within a hierarchy and that such a stance may have work-related consequences (Levy 2004).

The 'evidence' a woman refers to may include first- or second-hand knowledge of particular clinical situations and outcomes, which, while statistically irrelevant, have a powerful impact for that woman on an individual level. However, some of the 'evidence' available (and there is no shortage of books, magazines and online material) sometimes appears less than well-informed. In her critique of the book *Babies for Beginners*, Hunt (2004: 279) refers to the author's claim that 'giving breast milk will have no influence on a child's future health and therefore bottle- or breast-feeding is merely a matter of parental choice'. The vast amount of data on the benefits of breastfeeding can be ignored, it seems. A book still popular in the USA called *The Girlfriend's Guide to Pregnancy* (Iovine 1995) discusses the benefits of elective caesarean section, and states 'you will enter the hospital in a fairly calm and leisurely fashion, and (the doctor) will extract your baby through a small slit at the top of your pubic hair.' This apparent trivialisation of the procedure can be criticised for masking the true nature of what is still major abdominal surgery (Wagner 2000).

MAKING DECISIONS

Midwives, as noted above, are often in a position where they are asked to provide information and even advice, and are also expected to act as the woman's advocate (cf. Warriner 2003,

Levy 2004). On the one hand, if women are well informed and are deemed to be capable of making decisions on their own behalf, they should not really need someone else to speak for their cause. The reality is that such decisions are not made on a level playing field: much of the information and knowledge is held (and its nature determined) by healthcare professionals. The RCM (2000: 8) has noted that 'women tend towards compliance if they are led to believe that they or especially their baby is at risk'. This does raise the issue of power relations when discussing matters or making decisions. Cruickshank (1999: 143) points out that 'it is not a shameful or dishonorable thing to possess special knowledge and judgment. In fact, one could argue that is what being part of a "learned profession" is all about.' In a legal sense, of course, the paradox remains: it is well established in Britain that providing a woman is mentally competent she can make decisions concerning her care, and that to take clinical steps to override such decisions would have serious consequences, notwithstanding professional or moral objections to the woman's decision. O'Boyle considers the question of consent in Chapter 3.

Much is made of how decisions should be informed by sound evidence. The MIDIRS (the Midwives Information and Resource Service, an educational charity set up in 1985 to be a source of information for midwives and others involved in maternity care) *Informed Choice* leaflets (MIDIRS 2005) have been produced to provide practitioners and pregnant women with 'an objective appraisal of the best available scientific evidence relating to ... pregnancy, childbirth and postpartum. The Informed Choice topics include those specified in the Clinical Negligence Scheme for Trusts (CNST) Maternity Standards.' In referring to 'the best available *scientific* evidence' (my emphasis) there is an acknowledgement that the scientific paradigm predominates; individual narratives that gainsay an advocated approach may be a kind of evidence, but in terms of advising courses of action they do not count. In this quote there is also the admission that areas considered important in a medico-legal sense are critical. In a review of the impact of these leaflets, Wiggins & Newburn (2004: 161) concede that there is still some way to go in terms of influencing decision-making, and they conclude that 'women's choices during labour and delivery remain limited'.

All of this discussion relates to a context in which, as noted earlier, maternal and perinatal mortality rates are much lower than they once were. In western societies we are privileged to be in a position where we can debate such things. While outcomes in childbirth should certainly never be taken be granted, it is instructive to be reminded that there are countries where such outcomes are frequently catastrophic. A sombre definition of maternal risk is given by the World Health Organization (1998): 'the probability of dying or experiencing serious injury as the result of pregnancy or childbirth.' In advocating use of its partograph, the World Health Organization (1994) notes that this simple tool can be used to save lives (this comes back to the epidemiological model). The application of 'alert' and 'action' lines are designed to prompt saving interventions, and have led to what is known as 'active management of labour', in which the woman's scope for making decisions is curtailed by predetermined hospital policies. While criticised for being unnecessarily deterministic (Shepherd 2003), this approach remains in place in some Western countries.

PROTOCOLS

This brings us on to the matter of protocols, which have come to play a central feature in this debate. Once again, this process is not restricted to healthcare. Regulation and guidance are significant factors in most areas of employment, and there is some dispute as to its proper role. The Better Regulation Task Force (established in 1997, this is an independent body that advises the UK government on matters relating to regulation) warns against what it calls 'regulatory creep' – the restriction of activity through fear of being criticised or sued:

> The language used in guidance can also add to the confusion. Frequent use of the word 'should' tends to make those using guidance feel that they have no choice but to follow it to the letter

(BRTF 2004: 17).

The same argument is present within health-care, where practitioners can feel constrained by protocols (Symon 2001), despite the National Institute for Clinical Excellence stating that guidelines and protocols should not be followed blindly – they are recommendations for action, not instructions. (NICE, a Special Health Authority set up within the National Health Service, operates only in England and Wales. In April 2005 it became the National Institute for Health and Clinical Excellence (still to be known as NICE).) They reassert that practitioners are accountable for what they do and for what they do not do, and that while guidance is thought to be robust and based on a consensus of medical opinion, applying a protocol uncritically (akin to 'just following orders') is no defence. The development of protocols can be criticised for being 'top-down' – in other words produced by professionals for professionals, and without consideration of those directly affected by clinical care. Ideally, they should be written in consultation with service users. Sensitively applied, they should be non-directive and inclusive, so that a pregnant woman is consulted and her wishes taken into account when discussing management options.

Midwives and obstetricians do not work in a vacuum: clinical practices are determined by other factors such as codes of practice in addition to local and national protocols. While there should certainly be no 'one-size-fits-all' approach in applying protocols, it can be questioned whether they are always applied to individual cases. Much seems to depend on the person discussing matters with the woman concerned. Mead's (2003) study of the culture of different units found that midwives tended to be socialised into a unit's way of thinking:

those working in units that had higher intervention rates generally had a higher perception of risk for women who were in fact suitable for midwifery-led care. This appears to reduce the scope for choice for a pregnant woman in such a unit, for it seems that she cannot rely on the midwife being sympathetic to a request to be treated as low risk.

It may be more helpful to use the term 'decision aid' than protocol/guideline/policy, not least because the latter terms are inconsistently defined and applied. According to Roberts et al (2004: 1–2):

> Decision aids are designed to assist patients and their doctors in making informed decisions using information that is unbiased and based on high quality research evidence. Decision aids are non-directive in the sense that they do not aim to steer the user towards any one option, but rather to support decision making which is informed and consistent with personal values.

This certainly appears to sum up the most reasonable approach in the context of maternity care, where the expectation is that we are dealing with healthy and mentally competent adults. There is scope for a consideration of the available evidence (although research evidence is necessarily partial), including the woman's own views, and there is usually time for different options to be weighed up. This does require that the various options for care are discussed at a time when there is no pressure to make decisions; in most cases this applies to most of a pregnancy. This brings into question the risk categories used in maternity care, how and when they are applied, and how they interact with choice.

RISK AND CHOICE

There is an argument that modern governments use fear in order to sustain their authority (Furedi 2004), and this argument can be extended to healthcare providers: in their desire to maintain professional authority, the claim (implicit or explicit) is made that only by acceding to technocratic or professional authority can a woman maximise her chances of avoiding catastrophe.

The changing face of maternity care provision has led to a streamlining process, by which women are often placed into a risk category at the time of booking. Those deemed suitable for midwife-led care may be categorised 'low risk'; those with certain 'risk factors' may correspondingly be deemed unsuitable for such care, and consequently labelled 'medium' or 'high risk'. While a woman who is 'low risk' at the start of the pregnancy may be re-labelled as 'medium' or 'high risk' later on, very rarely does this process work in the other direction. Almost always the risk label is applied rather than requested – in fact there is some evidence that women tend to perceive themselves as being lower risk than professionals do (Stahl & Hundley 2003). If this categorisation is genuine, then there would appear to be an inverse rule, whereby a woman's ability to exercise choice diminishes as her imposed risk category increases. However, this may depend on the nature of the choice the woman would like to make – some women may request more monitoring or interventions than would appear to be warranted by their 'risk label'. There are of course additional considerations for health service planners: some requests or choices may require additional resources (cf. Elwyn & Edwards 2001). There may also be ethical issues – elective caesareans, for example, do have an associated morbidity for both mother and baby.

Risk and choice can be painted as confrontational issues, as if pregnant women only ever wanted one type of care, and were only ever offered a different type. In reality, and given the generally good relationships that exist between most pregnant women and most healthcare practitioners encountered during the course of their pregnancy, the matter may not be as oppositional. While we must guard against concluding that women are truly satisfied with the care they receive – Hundley & Ryan's (2004) study found that women tend to say they want what they're offered – it is hard to be certain how much dissension there

truly is between women and midwives or obstetricians.

Place of birth is a critical issue, and many practitioners may be unhappy at the prospect of a woman with identified 'risk factors' (however these were derived) planning childbirth anywhere other than in a fully equipped unit. This is considered by Smith in Chapter 7 and O'Connor in Chapter 10. From the woman's point of view it may be difficult to press home her desired choice if told that emergency backup may not be available for a home birth or even one within a 'low-risk' unit. The inverse rule seems to apply here. At the next rung on the ladder, the same woman may be told she is 'not suitable' for her local 'low-risk' unit. If she is keen to avoid routine monitoring and the increased likelihood of clinical interventions that are associated with 'high-risk' units, does she have any more choice? Is she, as Adams (1995) might have it, simply expressing her own thermostatically-determined view of risk?

These scenarios raise a number of issues, such as how risk is perceived; how it is analysed; how choices are made; and how tensions are resolved when there is disagreement. It also begs the question of how reflection is used by those involved in these discussions to inform future decisions. These issues, which must be seen against the backdrop of wider societal trends, are considered in this book from a range of angles, including international perspectives.

References

Adams J 1995 Risk. UCL Press, London

AIMS (Association for Improvements in the Maternity Services) 2004 Birth after caesarean. AIMS, Surbiton

Anderson T 2004 The misleading myth of choice: the continuing oppression of women in childbirth. In: Kirkham M (ed) Informed choice in maternity care. Palgrave, Basingstoke

AS/NZS (Australian Standard/New Zealand Standard) 2004 Risk Management (AS/NZS 4360). Standards Australia

BBC 2005 Deadline for dangerous food dye. Online. Available: http://news.bbc.co.uk/1/hi/health/4290975.stm 23 Feb 2005

Bellaby P 2001 Evidence and risk: the sociology of health care grappling with knowledge and uncertainty. In: Edwards A, Elwyn G (eds) Evidence-based patient choice: inevitable or impossible? Oxford University Press, Oxford

Bellaby P 2003 Communication and miscommunication of risk: understanding UK parents' attitudes to combined MMR vaccination. British Medical Journal 327: 725–728

BRTF (Better Regulation Task Force) 2004 Avoiding regulatory creep. Online. Available: http://www.brc.gov.uk/downloads/pdf/hiddenmenace.pdf

Clements RV 2001 Risk management and litigation in obstetrics and gynaecology. RSM/RCOG Press, London

Cruickshank DP 1999 Informed consent, patient choice, and physician responsibility. Obstetrics and Gynecology 94(1): 142–143

DH (Department of Health) 2004 The NHS improvement plan: putting people at the heart of public services. The Stationery Office, London (Cm 6268). Online. Available: www.dh.gov.uk/assetRoot/04/08/45/22/04084522.pdf

Doyle M 2004 Food recall process is called ineffective. Sacramento Bee, 30 Oct. Online. Available: http://www.sacbee.com

Edwards A, Elwyn G, Mulley A 2002 Explaining risks: turning numerical data into meaningful pictures. British Medical Journal 324: 827–830

EGAMS 2002 Expert Group on Acute Maternity Services Reference Report. Scottish Executive, Edinburgh. Online. Available: www.scotland.gov.uk/library5/health/egas.pdf

Elwyn G, Edwards A 2001 Evidence-based patient choice? In: Edwards A, Elwyn G (eds) Evidence-based patient choice: inevitable or impossible? Oxford University Press, Oxford

Furedi F 2004 The politics of fear. Spiked 28 Oct. Online. Available: www.frankfuredi.com/articles/politicsFear-20041028.shtml

Gabe J 1995a Medicine, health and risk. Blackwell, Oxford

Gabe J 1995b Health, medicine and risk: the need for a sociological approach. In: Gabe J (ed) Medicine, health and risk. Blackwell, Oxford

Godolphin W 2003 The role of risk communication in shared decision making. British Medical Journal 327: 692–693

Harrabin R, Coote A, Allen J 2003 Health in the news. King's Fund, London

Hewson B 2004 Informed choice in maternity care. In: Kirkham M (ed) Informed choice in maternity care. Palgrave, Basingstoke

HSE (Health and Safety Executive) 1999 Five steps to risk assessment. Online. Available: http://www.hse.gov.uk/pubns/indg163.pdf

Hundley V, Ryan M 2004 Are women's expectations and preferences for intrapartum care affected by the model of care on offer? British Journal of Obstetrics and Gynaecology 111(6): 550–560

Hunt S 2004 Review of 'Babies for beginners' by Jay R. White Ladder Press, Great Winbrook: MIDIRS Midwifery Digest 14(2): 279

Iovine V 1995 The girlfriend's guide to pregnancy. Pocket Books, New York

Johnson R, Slade P 2002 Does fear of childbirth during pregnancy predict emergency caesarean section? British Journal of Obstetrics and Gynaecology 109(11): 1213–1221

Kavaler F, Spiegel AD 2003 Risk management in healthcare institutions. Jones and Bartlett, Sudbury, Massachusetts

Levy V 2004 How midwives used protective steering to protect informed choice in pregnancy. In: Kirkham M (ed) Informed choice in maternity care. Palgrave, Basingstoke

Mead M 2003 Intrapartum care of women suitable for midwifery-led care: midwives' perception of their own and their colleagues' practice. Evidence Based Midwifery 1(1): 4–11

MIDIRS (Midwives Information and Resource Service) 2005 Informed choice. Online. Available: www.infochoice.org/

NHS MA (NHS Modernisation Agency) 2004 Midwifery-led care for low risk women in labour. NHS Clinical Governance Support Team. Online. Available: http://www.cgsupport.nhs.uk/Case_Study_Downloads/PDF/Maternity/PENS_Management_of_Women%20_in_Labour.pdf

Paling J 1997 Up to your armpits in alligators: how to sort out what risks are worth worrying about. Risk Communication and Environmental Institute, Gainesville, FL. (Paling palettes are available online at: The Risk Communication Institute website: http://www.riskcomm.com/paling_palettes.htm

Quilliam S 1999 Clinical risk management in midwifery: what are midwives for? MIDIRS Midwifery Digest 9: 280–284

RCM (Royal College of Midwives) 2000 Reassessing risk: a midwifery perspective. RCM, London

RCM 2003 Assessing and managing risk in midwifery practice. RCM, London

RCM 2005 Litigation: a risk management guide for midwives. RCM, London

Roberts CL, Nassar N, Barratt A et al 2004 Protocol for the evaluation of a decision aid for women with a breech-presenting baby. BMC Pregnancy and Childbirth 4(26) (20 December 2004). Online. Available: http://www.biomedcentral.com/ 1471–2393/4/26

Shepherd S 2003 Commentary on 'Active management of labour revisited: the first 1000 primiparous labours in 2000' by Bohra U, Donnelly J, O'Connell MP et al. (Journal of Obstetrics and Gynaecology 23(2): 118–120) MIDIRS Midwifery Digest 13(3): 357

SIRC (Social Issues Research Centre) 2000 Code of Practice/Guidelines on Science and Health Communication. Online. Available: http://www.sirc.org/publik/cop_guidelines_ j.html (see also www.sirc.org/news/ wising_up_to_scaremongers.html)

Smith AF 2002 Discussion of risk pervades doctor-patient communication (letter). British Medical Journal, 325: 548

Stahl K, Hundley V 2003 Risk and risk assessment in pregnancy – do we scare because we care? Midwifery 19: 298–309

Symon A 2001 Obstetric litigation from A-Z. Quay Books, Salisbury

Thornton H 2003 Patients' understanding of risk. British Medical Journal 327: 693–694

Wagner M 2000 Choosing Caesarean section. Lancet 356: 1677–1680

Wainwright M 2005 No napkins . . . elderly might eat them. The Guardian 13 April.

Warriner S 2003 Midwives: advocates or arbitrators? British Journal of Midwifery 11(9): 532–533

WHO (World Health Organization) 1994 WHO partograph reduces complications of labour and childbirth. WHO, Geneva, 7 June 1994 (press release)

WHO 1998 World Health Day Safe Motherhood. WHO, Geneva. Online. Available: http://www.who.int/docstore/world-health-day/en/pages1998/whd98_05.html

Wiggins M, Newburn M 2004 Information used by pregnant women, and their understanding and use of evidence-based Informed Choice leaflets. In: Kirkham M (ed) Informed choice in maternity care. Palgrave, Basingstoke

Wilson M, Symon A 2002 Clinical risk management in midwifery – the right to a perfect baby? Butterworth Heinemann, Oxford

Woloshynowych M, Adams S 1999 The perception of risk in obstetric care by obstetric healthcare professionals. Healthcare Risk Resource 2(3): 14–17

Chapter **2**

Healthcare's Hidden Risks: Identifying Vulnerability in Healthcare Systems

Brian Kennedy

'The truth is rarely pure and never simple'
OSCAR WILDE

ACKNOWLEDGEMENTS
Sincere thanks are due to Mr Wayne Gault, Mrs Pat O'Connor and Miss Donna O'Boyle for reviewing this manuscript and providing their forthright and valued opinions.

We live in a universe of choice, where our thirst for knowledge lights many paths through a landscape rich in opportunity. Unfortunately, every choice comes hand in hand with 'risk', an array of threats that must be identified, evaluated, controlled and ultimately accepted within a mature decision-making process. Initiative and innovation are rightly celebrated, but decision-makers must be awake to the concept of risk if they are to avoid quietly sleepwalking over the precipice. Hence we have seen the advent of corporate governance, as society seeks to balance risk and reward, and responsible managers work out how best to deal with risk and still profit from opportunity.

Consider the quantum leaps in healthcare that have been applied to the benefit of some parts of the world over the past decade or two. These advances hold the promise of outcomes that seem incredible to those from previous generations who remember darker days when medical optimism was less plentiful. Occasionally, however, promises are not fulfilled. Risk is the shadow of uncertainty that surrounds future outcomes, which are not always quite as predictable as we would like them to be. Risk management is a response to this, and can be considered to be an attempt to impose order, and increase the predictability of outcomes, by reducing future uncertainty. This chapter will try to identify the roots of that uncertainty by looking at workplace systems, the actions and motivations of those who work within them and the way in which the activity of those individuals is organised. As such, our brief journey takes a structural, rather than a personal, approach to analysing risk. Since maternity care is contained within the overall and much larger field of healthcare, it is necessary to look outside maternity care at times in order to explore the structures and theories behind risk management.

RISK MANAGEMENT IN HEALTHCARE

Not only have managers been challenged by the new risk-related questions posed by patients, regulators and governments, but so also have their clinical staff, members of stable professional enclaves, who have discovered that traditional clinical research and audit activity cannot in isolation entirely discharge their evolving responsibilities. In response to this, 'risk management' and 'clinical governance' have been high profile initiatives, albeit there has been a degree of variability in application at the coalface. Before looking at some of the underpinning principles of risk management, it may therefore be useful to briefly consider how risk management might typically look in the clinical environment.

Firstly, at the interface with the health service user, the clinician will manage risk by undertaking an assessment of the patient's condition, involving analysis of medical history, evaluation of risk factors, and agreement of objectives. This gives rise to a treatment plan that is designed to meet those objectives, by combating identified threats to the wellbeing of the patient, followed by a post-treatment monitoring regime designed to meet the needs of that patient.

Review of a range of outcomes, as opposed to individual patient episodes, is generally achieved through clinical effectiveness programmes that are designed to improve the efficacy of interventions. These test clinical hypotheses, and therefore represent a form of quality assurance very much complementary to risk management. Patient outcomes will either reinforce or challenge the existing scientific hypothesis, with data being aggregated and analysed in order to inform clinical processes and modify decision-making criteria.

Traditionally, this is the point at which clinical involvement in risk management, or quality assurance activity, has tended to fade away. However, Smallman (2000) in a non-healthcare context, described the concept of operational risk, which relates to threats and vulnerabilities arising from business processes, including behavioural challenges posed by staff. Interpreted in the context of healthcare, it certainly occupies some of the same ground as Clinical Effectiveness, but requires a systematic and analytical view of the entire process, requiring the input of not only clinicians, but also support functions.

The success of any activity, clinical or otherwise, relies broadly on people, materials, equipment, methods and environment. This further requires effective organisational planning, structure and culture in order to weave these threads into a discernible pattern. To draw out uncertainty, the practitioner must systematically deconstruct these levels of organisation to identify intrinsic vulnerabilities and potential threats. This enables control measures to be implemented, strengthening processes and rendering them less likely to fail. However, there will still be some residual vulnerability, and operational risk management offers the possibility of creating resilience in the form of back-up routines.

It is from analysis such as this that traditional problems become apparent, including: failure of induction training; inadequate monitoring and mentoring of new staff; ill-defined roles and responsibilities; ambiguous and conflicting procedures; poor leadership; professional boundary issues; communication failure; inability to learn from experience; blame culture; and inadequate equipment (Kennedy 2004). Unfortunately, these types of problems are often not identified prospectively within processes, but only emerge retrospectively from deep causal analysis following harm to a patient, or patients. In fairness, one of the reasons for this is that the analysis is time-consuming, which creates problems in a system already stretched for resource, with midwives and obstetricians having scant time for their existing workloads.

At a quite different level again, 'strategic' risk management informs the Board (the executive and non-executive directors of the hospital authority) of impediments which lie in the path of the organisation's stated objectives, including those that might affect the entire industry sector. While the eventual destination might already be dictated politically, strategic risk management helps fine-tune the route to get there. Relevant considerations may be technological change, economic concerns, environmental damage, demographic shifts, social expectations and the legal landscape.

Although it has been useful here to stratify risk management, in practice these distinctions may be somewhat blurred. Service redesign or business cases, for instance, will be dictated at strategic level by organisational objectives and political priorities, but operational risk management should also be deployed within the project to improve the effectiveness of implementation. The key message is that effective risk management requires practitioners to be willing and able to cut through traditional boundaries in order to gauge the effect of dependencies across support services and clinical hierarchies.

SYSTEMS AND UNCERTAINTY

Risk management rests on the basic concept of 'the system'. In its broadest sense, a system can be thought of as any collection of components that works in concert to channel energy, for instance (i) the cells of the human body, (ii) the plastic and silicon assemblies which together comprise a computer, or alternatively (iii) the midwives, obstetricians, anaesthetists, paediatricians, pregnant women, mothers, babies and others who combine in the clinical environment.

Unless the system is highly specified, there will be many different ways in which components can work together, and the outcome of an episode will depend entirely on the manner of these interactions. For instance, failure to inform the correct staff following a recognised indicator of obstetric complication could affect the ability of the team to deploy its skills when needed. Just as there will be a number of combinations by which components might interact, there will be a range of possible outcomes, some of which will be acceptable and others unacceptable. Within this model resides the very nature of uncertainty. In order to improve performance, or in other words ensure that the actual outcome is more often the same as the intended outcome, the practitioner must check that components are, firstly, individually reliable and, secondly, work well together.

Ambiguous or conflicting procedures are often identified as a significant risk issue but, within the context of the system, what does this actually mean? Procedures simply specify the role of each component, and the timing and manner of interactions between components. Faithful application of the correct procedure at the right time should initiate a particular chain of events and hence outcome, but the converse is also true: application of the wrong procedure, or misinterpretation of an unclear procedure, may set in motion an entirely unexpected sequence and could yield unintended outcomes.

In the face of such complexity, it is indeed useful that systems in different organisations and industries display similar properties. Toft & Reynolds (1997: 61) described this as 'isomorphic theory', the upshot of which is that healthcare providers can learn not only from their own experiences, but also from those of similar providers and even from organisations in other industries. Systems theory therefore underpins learning from adverse events, because it enables the transferability of lessons from one situation to another.

For practical purposes, the system must be ring-fenced with boundaries. This presents a thorny problem for analysts who may be planning activity or determining the reasons for under-performance. Ideally, the boundaries should encompass all 'relevant' components and processing activity, but in reality, the practitioner can only aim to balance an achievable model of the system, against the receding likelihood of low probability failures arising from factors omitted from that model. If we include too much within the system boundary then the analysis becomes unjustifiably expensive and perhaps unmanageably complex. However, if we are overly restrictive in the drawing of boundaries then there is a good chance that the analysis will be unreliable.

For instance, consider Toft's retrospective report (Toft 2001) investigating the underlying reasons for a fatal medication error. A highly restrictive view of the system might have confined analysis to the ward in question, thus setting boundaries relatively close to the adverse event. However, Toft's analysis indicated that failings existed in pharmacy also, justifying wider boundaries. In fact, Toft identified issues in a variety of areas: in document control, which is not only a local concern but a general management issue; in the process by which staff are inducted and mentored by the organisation; in the rotation system for junior medical staff; in the variation in systems throughout the National Health Service (NHS) in England; and also in equipment design. At every turn, tighter system boundaries would have confounded such analysis, although who can say for sure that there were no relevant issues outwith even those broad parameters selected by Toft?

LATENT DEFECTS WITHIN SYSTEMS

Self-evidently, not all vulnerabilities result in loss; some are detected and others are simply enveloped by the resilience of the organisation. However, errors and failures may also lie dormant within the system (Vaughan 1996). These dormant problems may exist undiscovered for years, then combine with other factors to produce loss. Reason (2001) describes these 'latent failures' as the outcome of high-level decisions, usually remote from the point of loss. Conversely, he suggests that 'active triggers' are the errors and violations committed by those who are close to the loss in time and space. In fact, these active triggers are often induced by latent defects harboured deep within the system itself.

Unfortunately, historical attempts to analyse failure have often focused on active triggers,

ignoring latent defects. This overlooks the role of senior management in service failure, and transfers blame to operators or practitioners who often have little or no power to alter the system, and who tend to inherit the impending losses created by flawed strategic or tactical decision-making. Midwives and obstetricians who attempt to communicate within rigid hierarchical frameworks that tend to block rather than facilitate effective communication will recognise this problem. Within this model, an important point to remember is that events are rarely, if ever, caused by a single failure or trigger (Reason 1990). Instead, they normally require multiple failures to occur at the same time.

It is not difficult to see that where event analysis focuses only on the active trigger and ignores the latent failures, many of the underlying problems just lie in wait for the next active trigger to set in motion a similar train of events.

Near-accidents that are caused by faulty designs or unsafe practices, but which are explained away as 'operator errors' are unlikely to produce organisational learning

Sagan (1993)

This is an important concept because incubation of latent, or underlying, failure is a theme which binds together much of the work on accident causation. It is central to the Disaster Sequence Model of Turner & Pidgeon (1997) and was also adopted within the broadly similar Systems Failure and Cultural Readjustment Model (SFCRM) of Toft & Reynolds (1997). The SFCRM incorporates three main sections: the incubation period where latent defects build up within the system; the trigger and the effects of loss expressed in terms of societal impact; and finally the process of learning.

Effective incident analysis techniques stress the importance of delving beneath the surface to identify underlying or 'root' causes of system failure, but the identification of latent defects is as relevant to prospective risk management as it is to retrospective analysis. Nonetheless, practitioners should remember firstly that there will be many underlying causes, and hence the idea of a single root cause is rather simplistic, and secondly that not all such causes will ever be identified. This is directly related to the problem of setting appropriate investigative boundaries, discussed earlier, not to mention the difficulties of prising apart complex interdependent sub-systems.

Within the labour process, several disciplines can be involved in what may be a complicated clinical situation, for instance a rapidly deteriorating cardiotocographic trace, with a decision being made to move to operative delivery. Concurrently, there may well be an underlying culture of poor communication between junior and senior obstetrician, or between the midwife, obstetrician and anaesthetist. The traditional route might well be to automatically blame one of these individuals. Without gainsaying individual responsibility, however, communication problems could in themselves result from the nature of the management hierarchy, inadequate staffing, lack of experience, inadequate technology or perhaps even poor design of facilities. Whatever the underlying causes, just when management plans need to be agreed and acted upon quickly, the inability of one party to communicate effectively with another may lead to tragic results. In how many maternity units is this problem lying in wait for a particular set of circumstances to occur? Sadly, if the underlying issues are not addressed, then the first tragedy will not prevent the second, nor the second tragedy prevent the third, until such root causes as can be identified are dealt with firmly and effectively.

NORMAL ACCIDENT THEORY

In view of this complexity, it is entirely reasonable to ask if poor outcomes are inevitable. Vaughan (1996) indicated that all possible means of avoiding failure should be investigated, but believed that poor outcomes will never be entirely prevented. Similarly, Perrow (1999) invoked the twin concepts of 'inter-activity' and 'coupling' to suggest that, with particular regard to systems incorporating modern technology such as nuclear power

generation, we can never hope to fully appreciate all potential sources of failure. He contends that serious adverse events are therefore certain to occur periodically. This is known as 'Normal Accident Theory'.

The first contention of this theory is that complex interactions make unforeseen reactions between system components more likely, indeed unavoidable (Sagan 1993). This means that components will have unexpected feedback loops and branches which link to other components in an unplanned way which, in so doing, destabilise performance to introduce an element of uncertainty.

The second element of Perrow's theory is 'tight coupling'. He contends that this operates in tandem with complex interactivity to make adverse events inescapable. In essence, tight coupling suggests that the system has insufficient buffers to permit interventions before a failure in one component has a domino effect on other components. If complex interactivity makes an accident more likely, then tight coupling makes it more difficult to recover from the failure. Perrow suggests that tightly coupled systems are recognisable by their time dependent processes, the strict sequential ordering of parts of the process, the limited means by which the system can achieve a successful outcome, and the degree of precision necessary to run the system. Within tightly coupled systems, systemic redundancy, or buffer, must be pre-planned and built into the system in advance, whereas loosely coupled systems offer a much greater chance of creating solutions in the midst of a crisis.

Labour provides an example of a fairly time-dependent, and potentially complex process, which cannot be halted to acclimatise staff with new routines in the midst of a spiralling crisis. As a result, appropriate fallback procedures, skills and the use of equipment must be rehearsed and pre-planned.

Reason (2001: 9) notes that some healthcare activities take place:

. . . within complex, tightly coupled institutional settings and entail multiple interactions between different professional groups.

This is extremely important for understanding not only the character and aetiology of medical mishaps but also for devising more effective remedial measures.

Complex interactions and tight coupling are therefore relevant to the healthcare environment, and may be an important factor in understanding the underlying causes of adverse events.

HUMAN ERROR

Since many of the components of our systems are human, then it is necessary to consider the role of the human factor within poor outcomes. Reason (2001) defines error simply as '. . . the failure of planned actions to achieve their desired goal'. In his seminal 1990 work on human error, he argues that error is the price which mankind pays for its ability to construct models and deploy rules that regulate behaviour and facilitate speedy solutions. He contends that when an individual believes that one of their existing solutions seems to fit well with a current problem then the rules associated with that solution are recalled and applied to the situation at hand in order to easily repeat successful past outcomes.

The nature of the decision-making process is integral to the emergence of error, and this is described by Reason's (1990) 'Generic Error Modelling System' (GEMS). The critical point of GEMS is that individuals seek solutions that are least taxing on the intellect, and only undertake tasks of a more cognitively stressful nature when they absolutely have to do so. In practice, this means that individuals will seek routine solutions from their existing repertoire of rules, and only if this cannot be achieved will they attempt to create novel solutions. Consider this in terms of protocols, which are designed to create a library of routines, removing the variability associated with individual decision-making within commonly encountered situations. Unfortunately, misapplication of a procedure, perhaps because the problem is rather more novel than at first

appreciated, will in itself result in a poor outcome. These rules therefore have to be designed, introduced and applied with great care.

Reason identifies three forms of unintentional error, and three forms of intentional violation. The first type of unintentional failure occurs during the execution of routine tasks and appears as subconscious slips and lapses, which are usually associated with failures in recognition, attention, memory or selection, and may arise as a result of change (Reason 2001). It is well established, for example, that practitioners may err due to simply misplacing a decimal point, particularly concerning neonatal drug dosages (Chappell & Newman 2004). When these types of slip occur, the practitioner has the correct solution in mind but simply fails to carry it out properly.

The second and third forms of unintentional error are collectively known as mistakes. These occur during planning and problem solving, rather than merely routine task execution. One of these mistakes is associated with the misapplication of existing rules, while the other occurs when seeking solutions to novel problems for which there are no available rules.

The emergence of error, although not its precise nature, is predictable where individuals are placed in situations where their experience fails to match the quality of the problems facing them, in other words they have an insufficient library of rules from which to select. Stringent supervision and monitoring of new staff – midwifery, nursing and medical – is therefore very important, for example where midwives take on junior doctors' work, particularly where formal planned training is poor and accountability is unclear. It is also worth pointing out that the healthcare sector is particularly susceptible to mistakes involving the misapplication of existing rules, due to subtle underlying variability in working practices that on the surface may seem similar. This potentially affects staff on rotation, or those transferring between healthcare providers.

Intentional violations are considered quite separately, with Reason arguing that these types of failure are associated with motivational rather than informational problems. He offers three categories of violation, each of which requires a different type of solution. The first of these is the routine violation that may occur when shortcuts seem convenient, such as omitting to wash hands as a matter of course between patients. The second violation takes place when individuals seek to optimise their own personal goals at the expense of organisational goals, for example perhaps failing to take time to communicate effectively at the end of a shift. Finally, there are necessary or 'situational' violations that seem to be the only option available due to the apparent inappropriateness of existing rules for the situation at hand. Unfortunately, violations can be doubly problematic, as practitioners may feel obliged to conceal their actions, and deviance then becomes subsumed and normalised within day-to-day activity, creating a latent defect within the system.

Finally, Reason suggests an important additional category of violation that, tragically, is not unknown within the healthcare environment. This is 'sabotage', where the intention is to cause damage, the result of which may be fatal as in the well-reported cases of Shipman and Allitt.

HIGH RELIABILITY THEORY

Whereas Normal Accident Theory takes the view that occasional accidents are inevitable, High Reliability Theory promotes a more optimistic message. It suggests that organisations can build looped systems that successfully compensate for human frailty, and holds that the organisation as a collective is potentially more rational than its individual human actors could ever hope to be. Sagan (1993) pointed out that highly reliable organisations tend to have clear goals and strong structures. Furthermore, they attempt to block environmental influences and define the boundary of their system with some precision. From various studies, Sagan identified four key characteristics of allegedly highly reliable organisations.

Firstly, leaders have to be committed to safe and reliable operations, which must in fact

be an objective of every individual working within the organisation. Despite the tension between (i) safety and (ii) production or throughput goals, highly reliable organisations will set aside short-term gain for extreme reliability.

Secondly, highly reliable organisations create 'redundancy' within the system. This simply refers to the creation of extra capacity in the form of secondary back-ups that can take the strain if the primary system component should fail. However, planned redundancy can be enormously expensive, which is one of the reasons quoted by Sagan (1993) for stating that highly reliable organisations require leaders who are committed to reliability and safety.

The issue of redundancy is particularly relevant for the healthcare sector where the prevailing pressure is to make limited staff and equipment stretch ever further. Where there is no redundancy, safety margins are extremely unforgiving and the organisation can be expected to experience periodic failure. This was illustrated by a quote from the *Daily Telegraph* (2002), where an NHS chief executive lamented that his biggest problem emerged from '. . . running an organisation which runs permanently so close to its limits'. He went on to state, 'I am not surprised the system keeps breaking down'. Even where redundancy is planned into the system, there will eventually come a temptation to use that extra capacity for primary activity rather than to provide the safety margin that was actually intended, increasing the prospect of failure. Consider the matter of high bed occupancy rates which have, in certain respects, been shown to increase patient risk.

Sagan's third pillar of High Reliability Theory is the ability to decentralise to promote a speedy local response to problems by those best placed to deal with them. If this is to work effectively, it requires common values and the intense socialisation and education of employees to strive for safety in their local decision-making. Commitment to rehearsal and training is essential, which can have hefty resource implications, although there are instances of interesting practice in healthcare, as offered by Thompson et al

(2004) who detail the benefits of simulated eclampsia drills.

Finally, High Reliability Theory places great store by organisational learning, particularly by trial and error. Spear & Bowen (1999) conducted a detailed study into the reasons for the success of the Toyota automotive production process, and found that one of the critical issues was the commitment to continuous improvement at the lowest possible level in the organisation, through rigorous hypothesis testing stimulated by real-time performance data.

Despite the seductive simplicity of Toyota's approach, it seems likely that such measures are easier to implement in the relatively linear sequencing of an automotive factory than in a complex and dynamic healthcare environment. Effective learning of course requires sound information, which is partly why the Toyota system was so successful. Unfortunately, the origins of accidents in more complex systems may be numerous and partially indeterminate, which could lead to revisionist reconstruction of the event in such a way that merely concurs with pre-existing notions. Nonetheless, healthcare organisations are making significant strides in relation to learning from adverse events, but there is still room for improvement in reporting rates and the effective use of both quantitative and qualitative data.

Practitioners must also bear in mind that risk is a political concept, and failures are therefore fundamentally political events. Olsen (2000) believes that disasters tend to strip the organisation of its protective layers and lay bare its true values and processes. This leaves individuals feeling vulnerable, which in turn leads to blame, secrecy and cover-up, creating a confounding effect on the organisation's ability to learn from adverse events (Horlick-Jones 2001, Johnston 2001, Leape 2000; Reason 2001, Sagan 1993). In fact, Weir (2001) suggests that evidence about failure is normally regarded as at least subversive, if not overtly damaging. It is therefore wholly unsurprising that some organisations circle the wagons as a knee-jerk reaction to defend whatever integrity still remains within the system.

ANALYTICAL TOOLS

Having established that risk management begins with the concept of the system, practitioners still need effective analytical tools to take risk identification forward in a practical and methodical way. Most readily to hand are basic aids such as SWOT analyses (i.e. Strengths, Weaknesses, Opportunities, Threats) which can be used to strip out inherent risks within the system, and ascertain the external events that might affect its stability. This simple form of analysis also permits the practitioner to add value through linkages between, firstly, strengths and opportunities and, secondly, weaknesses and threats.

More sophisticated analytical tools have been developed in the manufacturing industries, with thus far limited cross-over into healthcare. In particular, 'Hazard and Operability Studies' (HAZOP) were developed to look at deviations in system performance, generally in industrial plant configurations. This is a two-way qualitative process which starts with identification of potential deviations within the system, based on pre-defined guidewords (e.g. too much flow, not enough flow, wrong type of input, etc.). HAZOP teams then look at not only the potential causes of each deviation but also the consequences (hence a two-way process), together with review of existing precautions and creation of action plans.

Failure Modes and Effects Analysis (FMEA) is another qualitative approach which can be used either stand-alone, or to complement a prior HAZOP. FMEA focuses closely on potential component failure and the subsequent consequences for the entire system. It is well-suited to taking into account human factors as well as hardware and software failure, and can be deployed in a healthcare environment. Cavell (2004) outlined an approach to reduction of medication error using an FMEA variant.

While FMEA and HAZOP are both essentially qualitative tools, Fault Tree Analysis (FTA) offers the possibility of quantitative outputs, assessing likelihood as well as describing consequences. FTA begins with identification of a 'top-event', such as the potential failure of a particular process or possible patient harm of some description. The contributing failures are then linked by logical 'and/or' gates and a tree is constructed, with the top-event at the apex and the potential root causes at the base. This approach demonstrates well the appearance of multiple failures within most adverse events. Fault trees are not solely a prospective tool (i.e. before an accident), but can also be retrospective (i.e. following an accident), and healthcare analysts often use simplified forms of FTA in root cause analysis.

Similar to FTA in its diagrammatical approach is Event Tree Analysis (ETA). Event trees are not concerned with causation but rather test the resilience of the organisation's control measures through analysis of accident sequences following the initiation of an adverse event. By tracing the organisational protections in place, and the probability that they will operate effectively, the event tree takes shape and provides a quantified list of potential outcomes from the initiating event. These will usually range from likely outcomes where the event is controlled and loss is minimal, through to less likely outcomes where the effects are catastrophic due to the failure or absence of safety systems.

CONCLUSION

Practitioners embarking on a programme of risk management must thoroughly understand the mechanics of the system in order to identify latent defects that may give rise to loss. Nonetheless, it is difficult to avoid the conclusion that the complicated and tight-knit nature of modern systems might render poor outcomes occasionally inevitable. Despite this, there are areas where, with sufficient resource, expertise and creativity, improvements are possible. In particular, High Reliability Theory has much to add to the debate on creating more reliable organisations, but its key weakness is maybe the illusion of control encouraged by an overly deterministic closed system approach. Of course, theory is of little tangible benefit to practitioners if it

cannot be usefully deployed and a number of practical approaches are available to shine a light on healthcare risk. Unfortunately, uptake has been gradual and operational risk identification and analysis is often less rigorous than might be expected in a potentially high hazard environment.

References

Cavell G 2004 Using failure mode and effects analysis to reduce medication. Healthcare Risk Report, November

Chappell K, Newman C 2004 Potential tenfold drug overdoses on a neonatal unit. Archives of Disease in Childhood Fetal and Neonatal Edition 89: F483–F484

Daily Telegraph 2002 The Chief Executive. 15 Jan. Online. Available: http://www.telegraph.co.uk/health/main.jhtml?xml=/health/2002/01/15/hnhs115.xml

Horlick-Jones T 2001 The problem of blame. In: Hood C, Jones D (eds) Accident & design. UCL Press, London

Johnston AN 2001 Blame, punishment and risk management. In Hood C, Jones D (eds) Accident & design. UCL Press, London

Kennedy BM 2004 The influence of latent systemic factors on adverse events in healthcare. Healthcare Risk Report 10(9), September

Leape LL 2000 Reporting of medical errors: time for a reality check. Quality in Healthcare 9: 144–145

Olsen R 2000 Towards a politics of disaster: losses, values, agendas, and blame. International Journal of Mass Emergencies and Disasters 18(2): 265–287

Perrow C 1999 Normal accidents: living with high risk technologies. Princeton University Press, New Jersey

Reason J 1990 Human error. Cambridge University Press, Cambridge

Reason J 2001 Understanding adverse events: the human factor. In: Vincent C (ed) Clinical risk management: enhancing patient safety. BMJ Books, London, p 9–30

Sagan S 1993 The limits of safety. Princeton University Press, New Jersey

Sexton JB, Thomas EJ, Helmreich RL 2000 Error, stress, and teamwork in medicine and aviation: cross-sectional surveys. British Medical Journal 320: 745–749

Smallman C 2000 What is operational risk and why is it so important? Risk Management: An International Journal 2(3)

Spear S, Bowen HK 1999 Decoding the DNA of the Toyota production system. Harvard Business Review, Sept-Oct: 96–106

Thompson S, Neal S, Clark V 2004 Clinical risk management in obstetrics: eclampsia drills. BMJ.com, 328: 269–271 (31 Jan)

Toft B 2001 External inquiry into the adverse incident that occurred at Queen's Medical Centre, Nottingham, 04 January 2001. Department of Health, London

Toft B, Reynolds S 1997 Learning from disasters: a management approach. Perpetuity Press, Leicester

Turner B, Pidgeon N 1997 Man-made disasters. Butterworth-Heinemann, Oxford

Vaughan D 1996 The Challenger launch decision: risky technology, culture and deviance at NASA. University of Chicago Press, Chicago

Weir D 2001 Risk and disaster: the role of communications breakdown in plane crashes and business failure. In Hood C, Jones D (eds) Accident & design. UCL Press, London

Further Reading

Arthur H, Wall D, Halligan A 2003 Team resource management: a programme for troubled teams. Clinical Governance: An International Journal 8(1): 86–91

Bennett S 2001 Human error – by design? Perpetuity Press, Leicester

Clothier C 1994 The Allitt Inquiry. HMSO, London

Degeling P, Maxwell S, Kennedy J et al 2003 Medicine, management and modernisation: a 'danse macabre'? British Medical Journal 326: 649–652

DH 2001 Doing less harm, version 1.0a. HMSO, London

Douglas M 1990 Risk as a forensic resource. Daedalus 119: 1–16

Gallagher EJ 2002 How well do clinical practice guidelines guide clinical practice? Annals of Emergency Medicine 40(4): 394–398

Gosbee J, Lin L 2001 The role of human factors engineering in medical device and medical system errors. In: Vincent C (ed) Clinical risk management: enhancing patient safety. BMJ Books, London, p 301–318

The Guardian 2003 Key points of the Shipman Reports. 21 Aug. Online. Available: http://www.guardian.co.uk/print/0,,4712054–103690,00.html

Thomas EJ, Brennan TA 2001 Errors and adverse events in medicine: an overview. In: Vincent C (ed) Clinical risk management: enhancing patient safety. BMJ Books, London, p 31–43

Chapter **3**

Why Informed Consent is Important in the Exercise of Maternal Choice

Donna O'Boyle

INTRODUCTION

The delivery of modern healthcare is underpinned by multi-faceted responsibilities to individuals, society, and also professional bodies. This chapter describes the approach within the UK, however the legal principles discussed here are equally transferable to any common law jurisdiction, and the ethical principles transcend any geographical limitations. Individuals want the care that best suits their needs; society demands that we do so within a legal framework; and professional regulatory bodies aim to ensure that we adhere to professional and ethical codes. At first glance, there would appear to be few areas where concordance in all of these principles cannot be reached. However, look a little deeper and it can easily be seen that there are in fact many instances where tension arises: the plea for an individual to die a death at the time and in a manner of their choice conflicts with the legal stance on opposing euthanasia; the contested right to continued treatment of children where further clinical intervention has been deemed futile by medical staff; and the current debate on the ethical aspects of the use of cloned materials. These are simply a few examples to which contemporary society will no doubt add as new treatments emerge and societal expectations rise. However, they are also scenarios that have recently given rise to legal challenge, and although all very different, they have at least one common element: consent. Consent in contemporary healthcare does not simply mean asking someone's permission to medically touch; it is this of course but it is also much more. Maternity care presents the opportunity for very intimate and profound intervention, yet some commentators (Levy 1999, Robertson 2003), when discussing the application of consent in maternity care, claim that women are effectively being denied the right to the full spectrum of potential care options. Whether this alleged practice is deliberate, a remnant of a bygone paternalistic approach, or an attempt to influence the woman in a genuinely held belief that the most appropriate options are being presented in her best interests, it is worthy of further examination.

With consent as an integral element of healthcare, there exists a plethora of guidance to support us in this quest. Contemporary medical ethics bid us to give respect for autonomy – the right to self-determination. Professional organisations guide us in expected behaviour when treating an individual. Further, the rights and responsibilities that healthcare staff must recognise are contained within various legal statutes and decisions at common law.

However, it appears increasingly problematic for healthcare staff to understand and apply all of these elements in practice. There are several published studies (Aveyard 2005, Karpouzie et al 2005, Marshall & Baker 1999, Plant & Scholefield 1999) that highlight the incomplete understanding of healthcare staff in the realm of consent. Perhaps of more importance, is that many staff labour under the misconception of their interpretation of what the law does and does not allow them to do. When staff 'don't know what they don't know' it can be difficult to uncover flawed decision-making until actual harm arises. The incidence of complaints involving consent as the main element have risen steadily, and the Health Service Ombudsman's 2003 Report (HSC 2003) highlights the failure of patient-centred care and the breakdown in communication as an important, and worryingly, novel category. There is little to indicate that there will not be a corresponding number of dissatisfied women who seek redress through the civil legal system for unlawful treatment based on an incomplete consent process which has given rise to harm in the realm of maternity care.

In addition, there are two particular elements facing the delivery of contemporary healthcare in the United Kingdom that potentiate the need for enhanced understanding in the application of the principles of consent. The first of these is the expanding professional portfolio of respective staff groups. The need has arisen, whether through political impetus or as a result of the drive to broaden the scope of professional expertise, for healthcare professionals to embrace new skills and enhance their own immediate professional sphere: the growth of Midwife-Led Units are one such example. Initiatives taken as a result of the Working Times Regulations, which has as one of its key objectives the limitation of the working times of junior doctors, are designed to improve patient safety. However, as often occurs with change, improving one set of circumstances may result in inevitable, and sometimes negative, ramifications for others. The predicted unavailability of junior doctors to provide suitable medical cover, means that of necessity other staff groups are now adopting jobs that were previously the sole domain of medical staff: midwifery staff will no doubt be familiar with assuming tasks and roles formerly only performed by obstetric and paediatric colleagues. This change in workload for groups of healthcare staff is not all being imposed by authoritarian or legal edicts however, and there is much enthusiasm among nursing and midwifery staff and other allied healthcare professions, to evolve and acquire new skills. Positive outcomes may include increased job satisfaction, improved recruitment and retention, and perhaps even short-term solutions to skills shortages, through this acquisition of skills. However, it also exposes staff that previously have not considered the need to seek formal consent to treatment, to the need for acquisition of relevant skills. Secondly, the increased knowledge of the general public in all areas medical has risen proportionally with access to portals of information, not only through the internet but also through mechanisms such as patient support groups.

Inquiries into the aftermath of situations such as those which arose in Bristol, Alder Hey, and more recently that of Shipman, have ensured that information has been placed within the public domain and has served as a catalyst to many changes, most notably Clinical Governance. It has also heightened awareness among the general public that healthcare can, and sometimes does, go wrong. Certainly, the public may be conversant about treatments and their outcomes, but they are also more knowledgeable in the realm of their expected rights, and the responsibilities of healthcare staff towards them. Accordingly the expectations of medical intervention and of the staff who deliver such care have risen markedly. Patient-centred care has the capacity to enrich healthcare, and provides many opportunities to consolidate and drive forward Clinical Governance, while fully involving patients as true partners in their own care. Staff therefore must ensure that they are conversant with both the needs of the patient and the legal requirements when obtaining consent and have the knowledge and mind-set to meet the challenges and the opportunities afforded by rising public expectations, and also the demands of modern healthcare delivery.

WHY IS IT SO DIFFICULT TO UNDERSTAND?

What then of the sources of information to guide and support the maternity care professions in gaining consent to treatment? There exist well-established principles of consent that have developed through the legal process, and have often been the subject of detailed ethical and legal debate. In order to help interpret these legal standards, codes of professional conduct from the regulatory bodies have evolved from sources of law, and further, the Department of Health in England & Wales has produced a substantive practical guide (DH 2005). However, there still clearly remain some difficulties for midwives, obstetricians and others in distilling out the relevant issues. Perhaps some clue exists in the approach to knowledge acquisition. Medicine and other healthcare subjects have traditionally been taught with a strong emphasis on science and rationality; and the expectation that staff should in addition understand the processes of law, apparently contradictory and sometimes illogical to those outwith the legal professions, written in a distinct language style that only lawyers seem to be able to interpret, can be really very frustrating. Add to that the oft-contrary decisions where a higher court can overturn an already decided case (where the initial decision appeared to the untrained legal mind to be perfectly reasonable), and one can perhaps begin to understand the barriers that exist to a common understanding between the legal and healthcare professions.

The existence of a plethora of relevant legislation, case law and the ever-changing legal landscape may perhaps appear too time-consuming, and frankly difficult, to facilitate meaningful interpretation of relevant legal principles for individual healthcare staff. Yet there are many who would claim that this is simply a smokescreen disguising the fact that there really are only a few basic principles of consent, which when coupled with a thorough understanding of the concepts of autonomy and capacity, will decrease the risk of a mis-match between healthcare responsibilities and legal expectations. It is the intention of this chapter to assist practitioners to apply these concepts to practical scenarios, including emerging or novel situations, with confidence, so that the needs of the individual are met, while ensuring safe and professional healthcare practice.

AUTONOMY

In order then to underpin consent law, it is necessary first to understand autonomy – the right of the individual to decide upon the integrity of his or her own body. Autonomy is a basic tenet of medical ethics (Beauchamp & Childress 1994, Edwards 1996): indeed it is this whole notion that provides the basis for the law of consent, and it is a right that is legally recognised and protected:

> *Every human being of adult years and sound mind has a right to determine what shall be done with his own body; and a surgeon who performs an operation without his patient's consent commits an assault . . .*
>
> (*Schloendorff* v. *Society of New York Hospital* [1914], per Cardozo J @ 125)

When a woman chooses to exercise this right by permitting the intentional invasion of her bodily privacy, in a medical sense, it does not imply that a healthcare practitioner then has carte blanche permission to treat anything she desires. The woman still retains overall control of her own body, and each and every intervention is subject to renewed permission to touch. That of course is not to say that the cumbersome process of signing a consent form is required (see further discussions below) on every occasion, however the individual must knowingly permit to any further intervention. Indeed the Nursing and Midwifery Council (NMC) has made clear its position on this:

> *Obtain consent before you give any treatment or care . . . you must respect patients' and clients' autonomy – their right to decide whether to undergo any healthcare intervention.*
>
> (NMC 2002)

Logically, if a woman has the right to permit medical intervention, then she also has the right to refuse, or change her mind about treatment. This can be particularly difficult for healthcare staff to understand, especially where they can clearly see the benefit of the proposed treatment. However, a competent individual is free to make decisions based upon her own values, which might not necessarily be those shared by others.

The right to decline treatment exists even if the outcome is an expected and understood likelihood of death. Further, this right to decline treatment does not depend upon an explanation of the basis on which the refusal has been made.

> *A competent woman, who has the capacity to decide, may, for religious reasons, other reasons, for irrational or rational reasons or*

for no reason at all, choose not to have medical intervention, even though the consequence may be the death or serious handicap of the child she bears, or her own death. In that event the courts do not have the jurisdiction to declare medical intervention lawful and the question of her own best interests, objectively considered, does not arise.

> (*Re MB (an adult: medical treatment)* [1997], per Butler-Sloss LJ)

The refusal of treatment by an adult who has the capacity to make a decision is binding upon all those who seek to treat that individual; to deliver treatment in the face of an autonomous decision would offend ethical, professional and of course legal sensibilities. The principle of self-determination is a fundamental right that forbids any interference with the physical integrity of an individual, unless permitted by and limited to, the informed consent of the individual.

TRILOGY OF CONSENT REQUIREMENTS

As with any complex task, there are fundamental elements that must be present to achieve a successful outcome. Consent is not a one-step task; rather it is a process, with several elements interdependent upon one another. If one is missing, then there can be no achievable final product. Valid consent in law requires that:

- it be given by a competent person
- the person must be adequately informed about the nature and purpose of what she is agreeing to
- the person should be acting voluntarily and not under the undue influence of another

Simply put: is the individual able, with sufficient understanding, and free from external pressure, to expressly state their intention as to the proposed treatment? In many cases the answer will be either black or white, however there are also many shades of grey within this realm. Categories such as children and individuals with mental illness attract the invocation of special rules, however the primary intention of any such legislation is to preserve the individual's best interests and exercise choice in pursuit of autonomy. Since neither children nor those with mental illness are immune from becoming pregnant, they must also be supported in exercising their chosen preferences and giving informed consent in relation to maternity care. In order that a logical approach to gaining informed consent is taken, each of these steps is described more fully below.

THE COMPETENT PERSON

Whilst autonomy is an inviolate right, the ability of an individual to express his or her decision can be affected if that person does not possess the necessary capacity to do so. Competency has been described as the gateway to decision-making and respect for persons and autonomy (Gunn 1994). The quest for a competent person begins and ends with the person whose bodily integrity is the subject of proposed medical intervention, and not their spouse, babysitter, teacher or close friend. The commitment to recognition of individual rights precludes the wholesale labelling of an individual to a particular classification or group, for instance: mental illness; mental incapacity; children. There will be those who suffer from mental health problems who retain full capacity, and yet others who do not. The assessment of capacity must recognise the individualised approach, and each case should be judged independently. Every person is presumed to have capacity to consent or to refuse medical treatment unless and until that capacity is rebutted, and the onus for proving so lies with the practitioner. Consider the position in an emergency where a pregnant woman has been rendered unconscious in a road traffic accident and develops vaginal bleeding – there is no possibility that this person is able to state her preferences, permit or decline any medical intervention. In this situation, the woman obviously is not in possession of the necessary capacity to assert her autonomy. However, there are many other

circumstances where the strength of capacity is less than clear, or indeed may fluctuate. Assistance in determining capacity may be found in the 1994 case of *Re C* (*Adult: refusal of treatment*), which although not based on a maternity example, has been subsequently cited with approval in the legal consideration of maternal choice, and in cases discussed further below. *Re C* gave rise to the following three-stage test. Can the patient:

1. take in and retain treatment information;
2. believe it;
3. weigh that information, balancing risks and need, to arrive at a decision?

The facts in *Re C*, while not reflective of maternal subject matter, nevertheless are illuminative, provide clarification and make for interesting reading: C was a 69-year-old man suffering from chronic paranoid schizophrenia, with profound persecutory delusions, who was detained at Broadmoor Hospital. He developed a grossly infected right foot, subsequently diagnosed as gangrene. Surgical opinion was that unless the leg was amputated, there would be progressive infection that would cause imminent death. C refused amputation, his persecutory delusions manifesting in the expression that any treatment was only offered in a calculated bid to destroy his life. He also believed that he was an eminent surgeon, expressing grandiose delusions of an international career in medicine during which he had never lost a patient, and articulated a complete belief in his ability to recover from this present illness aided by his strong belief in God. C could quite clearly retain and understand the information presented to him, which when assessed via his personal systems of belief, allowed him to arrive at a decision. Whether or not his medical attendants shared the same values and beliefs was held irrelevant. Despite his delusions, the Court was satisfied that C possessed the requisite elements to satisfy a test for competency, and that his right to self-determination had not been displaced. In espousing the three-stage test described above, the Court endorsed a step-wise approach to determining capacity that has been adopted as the standard against which determinations of capacity are measured. All three elements must be answered affirmatively in order that capacity can be ascertained.

The test of competency varies from one context to another, and extremes of age do not preclude the ability to exhibit capacity. Consider as an example a pregnant 14-year-old: maturity and intellect levels fluctuate between individuals, and therefore it is not possible to state with any certainty that every 14-year-old will be competent to make this decision; each person must be assessed individually. An individual may be competent for some purposes and incompetent for others at the same point in time. For many, the crux will be the irreversibility of the treatment proposed, and the graver the consequences of the decision, the greater a commensurate level of competence must be displayed.

There are other factors that may have an adverse bearing, albeit temporarily, on the capacity of an individual: confusion; shock; fatigue; pain; drugs – all or any of which may apply to a woman in labour. These may erode capacity; however there must be absolute confidence that any of these factors are operating to such a degree that they have completely overcome the ability to decide. In *Re MB (an adult: medical treatment)*, a woman consented to an emergency caesarean section delivery, however having a fear of needles, she refused to consent to the venepuncture necessary to collect preoperative blood samples and for induction of anaesthesia. In granting the doctors permission to carry out the required procedure, the Court was satisfied that fear had paralysed her will, and therefore destroyed her capacity to decide, citing with approval the test laid out in *Re C*. Where, as in this situation, an individual is unable to display the necessary capacity, the Courts will decide on the best interests of the individual, and will normally err on the presumption of life. This presumption however is based on the woman's life, and not that of the fetus. The interests of the woman prevail over that of the fetus; the fetus accrues no rights as an individual until it is born and has drawn a breath, protected in UK law only by the Abortion Act (1967).

ADEQUATE INFORMATION

A doctor or midwife must take reasonable care to provide women with information that is adequate in scope, content and presentation. Whenever possible, this information should be provided in a clear, jargon-free manner, using diagrams, models or written explanation. The NMC (2002) reinforce this message: '. . . all patients have a right to receive information about their condition. Information should be accurate, truthful and presented in such a way as to make it easily understood.'

Within this explanation, it is important to note that the practitioner is expected to answer truthfully any question that the woman may pose, which of course is an increasing possibility given the rising public availability of medical information. Therefore it is important that the practitioner is as fully informed and prepared for the meeting as is possible. If a question is asked that cannot be answered completely, then the practitioner has a professional responsibility to seek alternative sources of information or to refer the woman to a colleague who can fully answer her questions.

Necessary elements of the consent process that must be explained are:

- the purpose of the treatment and its expected outcome
- any alternatives to the proposed treatment
- an outline of the risks and benefits
- the consequences of not having the treatment

It is imperative to document the discussion of these points, and in a systematic and orderly fashion. Queries may arise several years after the actual clinician/patient interface, and the oft-quoted legal standard applies – 'if it wasn't documented, it wasn't done', therefore recall may at best be incomplete, and a court may be disinclined to lend weight to an unsubstantiated testimony. The decision in a recent case (*Hamwi* v. *Johnston* [2005]) highlights the importance of accurate and contemporaneous medical records. The situation concerned the birth of a gravely disabled child, and the mother argued that she had not been properly counselled by the antenatal consultant regarding the risks of amniocentesis, as a result of which, she declined to have the diagnostic test performed. Had proper counselling been available, she claimed that she would have undergone the test and considered termination of the pregnancy. The Court considered the use of a checklist and further annotation in the medical notes as compelling evidence that the appropriate counselling had in fact taken place.

Discussion of the risks attaching to a proposed treatment or investigation appears to exercise the mind of many clinicians. Any risk which is significant, and to which the woman would attach importance, must be disclosed. For many, this approach carries overtones of medical paternalism, for it seems to be left to the clinician to decide what risks are, and are not, worthy of mention. Conversely, great care should be taken in simply repeating by rote a long list of potential adverse risks, such as may be found in standard written materials. Not only might this unduly alarm the woman, it also precludes proper discussion of each of the most significant risks, and ultimately it does little to enhance the consent process. Perhaps of central importance is that each woman is assessed as an individual. Professional clinicians, through clinical and social history taking and examination of the medical record, are expected to know about the people for whom they care. Therefore, a 1 in 5000 risk of temporary blindness following the distillation of eye-drops might not be significant for someone who is to have these drops administered into one eye. Would you mention this risk? However, consider that your patient already has only one eye; the significance now assumes much greater importance. The risk has not changed, however, the outcome for this person may have, in that the realisation of this risk will have a consequence of greater magnitude, albeit temporarily. There may be parallels here with a woman who has reduced fertility or only a single functioning fallopian tube, and the possible unintended effect of a proposed treatment may therefore carry enhanced risks for this individual.

Care also must be taken in articulating the likelihood of risk. Not everyone understands ratio or percentage expressions, and therefore the challenge is to ensure that each individual has grasped the concept of the possibility of an adverse outcome or unwanted side-effect occurring. The recent professional conduct hearing of Professor Sir Roy Meadows at the General Medical Council heard how an analogy with winning the lottery was unwisely and unprofessionally made when describing the risk of multiple sudden infant death syndrome. There is a need to identify those risks that are significant, and to ensure that they are expressed in an appropriate manner and language to enable understanding at a level that addresses the woman's needs.

ACTING VOLUNTARILY

Individuals frequently face dilemmas for which support and guidance is actively sought, whether of an informal or formal nature: does this dress fit me? Do you think it's a good idea to go to the desert on holiday in July? Sometimes genuine guidance is being sought, and sometimes we are merely seeking confirmation of our own views. Depending upon the objectivity or the subjectivity of the supporter, different answers may well be given. The over-eager sales assistant may encourage you to buy something you know you'll never wear, while the good friend may say 'I know you; you'll find the desert too hot'. These situations in everyday life might be described as benign; if the dress doesn't fit, it can be returned. If the desert is too hot, I won't go again in July. One's own free will prevails and the guidance sought can be either accepted or discarded. In the context of consent, however, the extent to which influential opinion operates is very important. Some people will look to the healthcare professions for support in making a treatment decision, and the practitioner must resist the temptation to verbalise thoughts in parallel with their own feelings or experiences beyond that of giving objective advice as described above. Most people are normally capable of making a decision, but when subject to medical care some become vulnerable and dependent on healthcare staff. Scott et al

(2003) highlighted the differences in perception of information imparted from midwives and received by the women they treated. In addition, information was supplied on a range of choices deemed appropriate by the midwives but which in fact might not be the only options available to the women. Indeed Levy (1999) describes how midwives have been found to act as:

> ... gatekeepers of information generally guided by benevolent intentions but they controlled the agenda. Women were steered in the direction the midwife believed was appropriate and may have been offered choices freely, to disguise the fact that other choices were not available.

Practitioners should take steps to avoid coercion and duress, and note that failure to allow someone sufficient time to consider their decision and ask questions may constitute a form of duress. Midwives need to ensure that information has not only been received but also understood by the woman, so that maximum mutual benefit can be gained.

An interesting development in terms of a pregnant woman's right to exercise choice has recently arisen following a debate concerning the 'Midwifery Supplement' of the latest CEMACH report (CEMACH 2004). A section in this encouraged midwives to enlist the help of family, neighbours and religious leaders to encourage women to comply with treatment. Following representations from user groups (e.g. Robinson 2005) and intervention by the NMC, it has been recognised that this guidance might encourage coercion of a woman to acquiesce to treatment she might not necessarily choose for herself, and would mean the midwife breaching the Code of Professional Conduct in relation to the woman's confidentiality and autonomy. An erratum notice on the CEMACH website states:

> Chapter 18 – Issues for Midwives. Page 248, Recommendations Point 4 should read:
>
> ... In some cases this may require the development of more flexible antenatal care systems and access to medical services; for instance, it may help understanding of the cultural influences on a woman's choice for care to have close liaison with family friends or religious leaders. In these complex cases it is essential that the midwife has close contact with her statutory supervisor of midwives.

While friends and family most often have the individual's optimal health as their priority in giving advice, there have been occasions where such influence has been found to overbear the autonomy of the individual. Midwifery staff who bring pressure to bear on a woman, utilising any elements of culture, religion or family to do so, would do well to remember the lessons learned from the legal case of *Re T* (*Adult: refusal of medical treatment*), where a young woman required a blood transfusion following the stillbirth of her baby. Initially she consented to the blood transfusion, but then withdrew her consent after she and her mother (*'a fervent Jehovah's Witness'*) had a private conversation. *T* was not a Jehovah's Witness, and after she became unconscious her father and boyfriend sought a court declaration that it would be lawful for her to receive this life-sustaining treatment. The Court held that her mother had exercised undue influence on her daughter, to the extent that *T*'s free will had been overcome, and therefore *T*'s refusal of treatment was invalid. While *T* had fulfilled the test for capacity, and had been given enough information as to the expected outcome, alternatives and risks, she had failed at this final hurdle to fulfil all of the elements required to give informed consent. Jehovah's Witnesses are not the only religious group to reject certain elements of medical intervention, and care should be taken to ensure that such people are not marginalised or subject to special arrangements. As already stated, whether there is a religious reason or even none at all, adult capacitous people are at liberty to accept or decline any element of treatment offered.

THIS INDIVIDUAL HAS CAPACITY – WHAT NEXT?

A woman who is deemed to have capacity must be asked for her consent to any intervention.

This consent can be given either by implied consent, or by express consent.

Implied consent can be inferred by someone's behaviour or acquiescence:

The law requires that an adult patient who is mentally and physically capable of exercising a choice must consent if medical treatment of him is to be lawful, although the consent need not be in writing and may sometimes be inferred from the patient's conduct in the context of the surrounding circumstances.
(*Re T* [1992], per Lord Donaldson MR @ 649)

It is probably the most common form of consent encountered in the provision of daily physical care, however it can only be utilised in a very narrow range of situations. These are limited to interventions where there is a negligible risk of harm occurring as a result of the medical touching. For practical purposes, interventions such as blood pressure measurement or venepuncture may fit the clinical and legal scenario. However, the use of blood or tissue gained through venepuncture or during other interventions, such as tooth extraction, may not be subject to implied consent, especially if research or purposes other than general treatment are intended. Many lessons have been learned from the uncovering of illegal retention of organs, and caution should be exercised if there exists any possibility of alternative uses or storage of the tissue or of data arising from it. Contemporary considerations for midwives can be found within the drive to support access to antenatal human immunodeficiency virus (HIV) testing, and to further support women to make informed decisions in the management of their lives in the aftermath of an HIV-positive result (DH/RCM 1999).

Express consent is the more usual form of consent familiar to many practitioners. Its invocation is required whenever there is more than a negligible risk of harm occurring as an outcome of this intended intervention. A consent form, duly signed and dated by both practitioner and patient, after fulfilling the three steps of the consent process, and detailing the proposed interventions, is of course the gold standard. However, contrary to popular opinion, this does not have to be recorded on a consent form to be extant. Express consent may be given verbally or in writing, however its form is less important than the process that underpins it. If the patient has capacity, has been adequately informed and is acting free from undue influence, and gives consent to the proposed intervention, the healthcare professional need only record this within the medical record. Conversely, if the patient signs a consent form, but has not been subject to the process described above, then the consent form is worthless.

This scenario arose within the Bristol cardiac babies affair – many parents had in fact signed consent forms, however the lack of transparency in the process negated these signatures, which eventually held the Health Authority liable for damages as a consequence. Midwives have notably embraced the process of detailing within the medical notes the express consent of the labouring woman to vaginal examination, which is both a pragmatic and professional decision.

THIS INDIVIDUAL DOES NOT HAVE CAPACITY – WHAT CAN I DO?

Where an individual does not possess capacity, it is not to say that he or she cannot be treated. The law in England and Scotland at present is expressed differently, with the inception in 2000 of the Adults with Incapacity (Scotland) Act, although England has similar legislation under construction. However, suffice to say that patients who do not have capacity to express a choice can be treated under the doctrines of 'necessity', or of 'best interests'. Necessity requires that medical intervention is undertaken to save life or preserve health, usually in extreme circumstances such as are found in Accident & Emergency or paramedic situations. However, it is strictly limited to those urgent interventions deemed necessary to achieve the above goals.

A wider concept, and one which underpins the Adults with Incapacity (Scotland) Act, is that of 'best interests'. Best interests are wider than simply medical best interests, and include factors such as spirituality, religion, and any other relevant principles that govern the ethos and attitude to life of the person in question. There will be a weighing of factors such as benefits versus risks, and the consequences of non-treatment, pain and suffering. While we have already seen how in cases of doubt the Court will strive to preserve life, they have also considered that the right to die can be in an individual's best interests, most notably in the case of Anthony Bland (*Airedale NHS Trust* v. *Bland*) who, left in a persistent vegetative state after a hypoxic incident, was allowed to die after withdrawal of his feeding tube was legally sanctioned. In the maternity scenario, we have been left in no doubt that the only best interests to be considered are those of the potential mother, and not the fetus. Society's interest in preserving life must yield to the self-determination of the capacitous individual, and whether that be at the expense of the unborn, or of the clinician's professional, if perhaps idealistic view of the wonders of medical intervention, then so be it.

SUMMARY

Is consent really so difficult to master? Well-established principles of consent have developed so as to be comprehensive enough, with a little lateral thought, to be applicable to the majority of individuals. Whether parturient women, mentally handicapped, children, mentally ill, demented, unconscious or just unsure (and parturient women can be a combination of any or all of the above), the preservation of autonomy finds a comfortable bedfellow in contemporary UK law.

Interpretation of the principles of consent, when left to individual health organisations or even individual practitioners, may have introduced inconsistencies in the realm of choice and options for treatment afforded to individual women. Although internal processes may occasionally break down, necessitating a hasty attempt to secure consent, blanket statements in consent policies which preclude the taking of consent once an individual has received a pre-medication do little to recognise the concept of

individual capacity. While this may be a pragmatic organisational approach to ensure that patients are not routinely signing consent forms on a theatre trolley, it may unnecessarily limit treatment options for an individual who actually remains competent to decide, and in the realm of labouring women, pays scant attention to their latent ability to decide. Similarly, instructions that relate specifically to Jehovah's Witnesses do little to enable staff to comprehend the ability of *any* capacitous person to refuse treatment, regardless of their beliefs, religious or otherwise. Provision of standard information leaflets may provide false security for staff that they have discharged their duty to inform, and take little cognisance of the actual information needs of the individual. An investment in staff education may result in properly informed and knowledgeable staff, who can realise their potential in contributing to the professional and patient safety agendas.

Of necessity, this chapter has only been able to provide a brief insight into this interesting area of medical law. There is a clear body of opinion that pregnant women are being presented with treatment options conducive only to convenience for the practitioner, and that such conditioning is insidiously and consistently reinforced from initial contact with practitioners at prenatal classes (Robertson 2003). Indeed the perception that women are being given the opportunity for informed choice, would appear to be held exclusively by healthcare professionals, and O'Cathain et al (2002) describe a UK survey which revealed that many women held a diametrically opposite view. The empowerment of individual women via a comprehensive approach to information provision, together with an investment in staff education, may assist clinicians in fulfilling their ethical and professional responsibilities:

> *you are personally responsible for your practice. This means you are answerable for your acts and omissions regardless of advice and directions from another professional*
> (NMC 2002)

Whether in delivering standard healthcare, or engaging in the expansion of professional boundaries, practitioners must ensure that they are prepared to accept accompanying responsibility and accountability and fulfil their obligations to the women for whom they care. Both as professionals, and as potential clients of healthcare, we must ensure that we understand the elements of consent and can confidently apply them to our practice, and not simply limit available choice to that preferred, for whatever reason, by the practitioner. As members of the registered healthcare professions we have no choice, however it must always be remembered that health service users do.

Legal Cases

Airedale NHS Trust v. *Bland* [1993] AC 789 (HL)

Hamwi v. *Johnston and North West London Hospitals Trust* [2005] EWHC 206 QB

Re C (Adult: refusal of treatment) [1994] 1 WLR 290

Re MB (an adult: medical treatment) [1997] 38 BMLR 175 (CA)

Re T (Adult: refusal of medical treatment) [1992] 4 All ER 649

Schloendorff v. *Society of New York Hospital* [1914] 211 NY 125

References

Aveyard H 2005 Informed consent prior to nursing care procedures. Nursing Ethics 12(1): 19–29

Beauchamp TL, Childress JF 1994 Principles of medical ethics, 4th edn. Oxford University Press, New York

CEMACH (Confidential Enquiries into Maternal and Child Health) 2004 Why mothers die 2000–2002 – Report on confidential enquiries into maternal deaths in the United Kingdom. Online. Available: http://www.cemach.org.uk/publications.htm

DH 2005 Consent. Online. Available: www.dh.gov.uk/PolicyAndGuidance/HealthAndSocialCareTopics/Consent/fs/en

DH/RCM (Department of Health and the Royal College of Midwives) 1999 HIV testing in pregnancy – Helping women choose. Information for Midwives, HMSO

Edwards SD 1996 Nursing ethics: a principle based approach. MacMillan Press, Basingstoke

Gunn M 1994 The meaning of incapacity. 2 Medical Law Review 8

HSC (Health Service Commissioner) 2003 Health Service Ombudsman for England Annual Report 2003–04. HMSO, London

Karpouzie K, Daros CH, Elliot L et al 2005 Informed consent: a comparative study of Greek and British nurse preceptors' beliefs to informed consent. ICUS NURS WEB J 24: 1–12

Levy V 1999 Midwives, informed choice and power: part 1. British Journal of Midwifery 7(9): 583–586

Marshall JE, Baker PN 1999 Informed consent – legal and ethical issues. Healthcare Risk Report, July/August 1999: 12–14

NMC (Nursing and Midwifery Council) 2002 Code of Professional Conduct. NMC, London

O'Cathain A, Walters SJ, Nicholl JP et al 2002 Use of evidence based leaflets to promote informed choice in maternity care: randomised controlled trial in everyday practice. British Medical Journal 324: 643. See also: O'Cathain A 2004 Can leaflets deliver informed choice? In: Kirkham M (ed) Informed choice in maternity care. Palgrave Macmillan, Basingstoke

Plant N, Scholefield H 1999 Obtaining consent to treatment. Healthcare Risk Report, May 1999: 10–11

Robertson A 2003 Online. Available: http://www.acegraphics.com.au/diary/archives/000223.html

Robinson J 2005 Avoiding professional misconduct. British Journal of Midwifery 13(6): 360

Scott PA, Taylor A, Valimaki M et al 2003 Autonomy, privacy and informed consent 2: postnatal perspective. British Journal of Nursing 12(2): 117–127

Chapter **4**

The Instability of Risk: Women's Perspectives on Risk and Safety in Birth

Nadine Pilley Edwards and Jo Murphy-Lawless

INTRODUCTION

Midwives are trying to create more sensitised models of maternity care to help them support individual women in pregnancy and childbirth. Yet the settings in which midwives practise are dominated by concerns about risk, risk factors and risk avoidance. Definitions of risk and the determination of risk factors are seen as central to the provision of maternity care services and shape the guidelines and protocols under which midwives must work. Women, midwives, childbirth activists and educators continually tell us that there are severe limitations to the scientific thinking on risk and to what can be measured as being 'risky'. This is the core issue we want to address. We are not going to explore the issues of scientific efficacy and accuracy of individual protocols that stem from the risk factors that science identifies. This is because, as MacKenzie (1990) has written, the very notion that there can be scientific accuracy needs to be closely questioned. We will argue that the current obstetric scientific meanings of risk are deeply ambiguous and become a tool of disempowerment for women and midwives. What we also want to raise is the importance of 'seeing' risk in different ways, beyond the limitations of the scientific lens.

Hence the focus of this chapter is two-fold: to set out the current sociological debates about risk and science and to connect this thinking to the deep concerns that women have expressed about the way risk perception has adversely affected their care during pregnancy and birth. Women's accounts of their experiences help us to explore and explain some of the ambiguities associated with the notion of risk. We suggest that there needs to be a broader framework in which to consider risk from women's perspectives. If midwives can place themselves and the care issues they face in this broader framework, they may feel more equipped and confident in supporting women who are trying to make sense of the tensions they face between the practices they encounter, their own beliefs about risk and the kinds of decisions they want to make in their pregnancies and labours.

POSTMODERNITY: THE CHANGED MEANINGS OF RISK AND THE PROBLEM OF CHOICE

Sociologists argue that we have entered a new level of uncertainty: they describe a general sense in society of unease, anxiety and concern. They use different terms to describe this era: postmodernity, late modernity, reflexive modernity (Bauman 1992, Beck 1992, Giddens 1991).[1] Writers comment that this complex era is distinguished by the dwindling of the traditional social structures that we relied on in the recent past to protect us from dangers as we journey through life.

For example, the nuclear family and extended family were once seen as a kind of social protec-

tion for people who struggled in the face of deep poverty. We believed that they provided a buffer against material insecurity. But in a rapidly evolving postmodern period, the shape of the family has now expanded to include a number of different forms, of which the nuclear family is only one. Feminism has drawn attention to the patriarchal and often oppressive nature of the traditional family form and women have sought to empower themselves by moving away from unsatisfactory and even violent family relationships. Thus a woman might well now participate in several forms of family life, moving from being in a partnership to being a single parent during her life course. But she may also have to forgo the kinds of material support that used to come with the more traditional family form. Research tells us that the single parent female household is most at risk of poverty because the state and the labour market do not step in to adequately support women in such circumstances (Glendinning & Millar 1992, Benn 1998). Midwives can often see this effect on the women they care for.

Another example of a social structure that has undergone substantial change is organised religion. Traditionally, we believed that belonging to religious groups provided people with shared meanings and a shared purpose. Such membership also provided emotional security and, in times of hardship, actual charity to tide one over. This practice too has subsided in Britain. In many ways, we have shifted from a belief in fate and trusting in a supernatural power to help us through life's uncertainties to placing reliance on science. We now expect science to protect or limit our exposure to life's hazards and dangers, by relying on science and scientific methodologies to make clear to us what our probable risks are.

Paradoxically, we are also experiencing a greatly increased sense of risk as the old industrial society has made way for this late or postmodern era. On the one hand, science has provided us with many of the benefits we now take for granted, such as the significant advances in medicine, e.g. in organ transplantation. On the other hand, new risks and hazards (climate change, increased exposure to carcinogenic substances) have emerged as side-effects

---

[1] These terms are trying to describe a society that has moved on from the period of 'modernity'. Modernity was characterised by the industrial society and the stable nation state of the nineteenth and twentieth centuries and the processes of social change that accompanied industrialisation, such as increased urbanisation. Now, we have moved away from the simple phase of industrial society, where, for example, it was common to think of having a job for life. Terms like postmodernity, late modernity, and reflexive modernity are used to capture how we now live in a society shaped by factors such as intensified science and technology including information technologies; a gender revolution; a globalised economy; and less stable, more flexible employment patterns; more diverse living patterns; and global environmental hazards.

of the way science works in tandem with technology. Science has been spectacularly successful in helping to produce the technologies, goods and comforts that are part of the conventional way of life in economically advantaged societies, but the price we have paid has been the creation of new risks. Moreover, many people are also concerned that our current emphasis on material fulfilment, based on unlimited access to commodities and consumerism, has contributed to a deepening of other forms of poverty, such as emotional and spiritual poverty.

The sociologist Ulrich Beck (1992) has termed all these complexities the 'risk society'. He argues that each technological development brings with it a new set of possible disruptions and risks. We can see this in the current debate about the safety of mobile telephones and masts. And, because these new risks come from the progress of science and technology, we face a new kind of problem. As Bauman (1992) outlines, our problem is that science is both 'poacher and gamekeeper': it creates new technologies and then tells us that it can solve the problems of the new hazards it has created. When science and scientific authorities make this claim about problem-solving, they are also sending out another critical message. This is that science alone can be the judge about risk and that science alone can accurately measure what risk is in an objective rational way (Bauman 1992). In effect, it is hard to speak about risk except by using the language and reasoning of science.

Many of the mainstream medical practices to do with childbirth reflect this kind of thinking which saps the confidence women may have about the processes of pregnancy and birth. Yet as we will demonstrate below, many women see birth differently; for them pregnancy and birth are based at least as much on embodied and intuitive knowledge, as on scientific knowledge. Within this wider frame of reference, different perceptions of risk arise.

RISK, RESPONSIBILITY AND CHOICE

A troubling element about the 'risk society' is the need for the individual to respond to all the risks science defines. It is as if the 'risk society' demands that the individual should take all the responsibility of tending to her own health in order to continue to be socially and economically useful (Beck-Gernsheim 2000, Peterson 1997). Thus the reports that daily pour out from scientific establishments face us with new 'evidence' about risks and we are told that we need to make the 'right choices' about this evidence, to reduce our risk exposure. We not only have to respond, but we have to make our 'choices' about these 'risks' as private individuals. Our 'choices' are filtered through dominant social values of individualism and consumerism that have superseded the older social support system (which might be said to have included the family, religion, and trade unions and the welfare state). In this setting, 'choice' is a compromised decision where the individual must make the best of a complex situation in a society where there is a diminished sense of mutual support (Bauman 1998).

Birth is in a peculiar position in the 'risk society'. Women and their babies in advanced post-industrial societies are less likely than ever to die in birth, but the growth of technological, medicalised birth has brought with it a greatly expanded discussion and discourse about risk. Pregnant women are expected to accept what medical experts say about risk and its management, to accept that medicalised birth is what makes birth safer and to make their decisions and choices accordingly. What this means is that science and medicine have already mapped out what women's 'responsible' decisions should be in order to reduce risk.

The overall discourse on risk pulls relentlessly on women and midwives as they attempt to negotiate the seemingly proliferating numbers of risks that are now seen to surround birth and the methods and technologies science invents to deal with these risks. Women are asked to make their decisions in line with the conventional medical thinking about risk reduction. Yet it is clear to many women that their subjective capacity to define and respond to risk can often run at odds with the conventional obstetric protocols about risk management. Therefore, if women make decisions about aspects of their care during pregnancy and birth that do not match up with the conventional obstetric views of risk, their decisions may be seen as threatening to the conventional systems of birth management.

Obstetric medicine has been very successful in persuading the public to accept that it alone can improve birth outcomes by identifying, managing and safeguarding against risk in birth. We know, however, that there is a multi-layered problem of how such scientific thinking tries to isolate, investigate and treat 'risk factors'. Sociologists of science point to a core problem in that the logic of science is a 'relativist and probabilistic' one (Adam & Van Loon 2000: 4). So for complex reasons of power, this probabilistic logic is either converted into 'statements of certainty and fact' or the establishment restricts scientific analyses to an 'acceptable focus on all that is factual and quantifiable' (Adam & Van Loon 2000). In other words, from the outset, risk assessment strategies are a hedged bet. Moreover, in relation to birth, they simply do not appear to work (Enkin 1994, Strong 2000): 'the already apparent disadvantages of the obstetric approach have such large order of magnitude, that in any clinical trial it would be considered unethical to continue with the obstetric "treatment" ' (Schlenzka 1999: 175). And, risk assessment strategies can result in extensive morbidity (Downe et al 2001, MacArthur et al 1991, Wagner 1994, *Which? Way to Health* 1990).

In spite of such evidence and the fact that many women may be troubled when they are subjected to the practices of risk management, many decide that they must ignore their concerns and be grateful that their baby is healthy. This is linked to the capacity of the scientific model to persuade us not only to accept it as the only judge of what is risky, but also the judge of what is a moral decision. To contest or ignore its definition of risk is to be seen as immoral, so much so that women find themselves labelled as 'bad mothers' for refusing to accept its thinking. This logic is how obstetric medicine becomes so powerful that women are forced to engage with it irrespective of their views (Davis-Floyd 1992, Martin 1987, Murphy-Lawless 1998a, O'Connor 1992, Rapp 1999, Viisainen 2000).

THINKING REFLEXIVELY ABOUT RISK AND BIRTH

Making sense of the realities of women's individual experiences and decisions compared with the claims of obstetric science is deeply challenging, but very important work. When, through their birth stories, women come to reflect on their experiences, the decisions they made and the contexts of those decisions, their reflections form a strong critique, *a reflexive critique*, of the medical discourse on risk. This notion of 'reflexivity' is becoming an important dimension of the 'risk society'. Sociologists argue that reflexivity comes about when groups and individuals other than expert scientists begin to reflect on how risks are produced and what their effects are. This is the start of a critical debate when scientific claims are questioned by people outside science and whom science would see as non-experts (Beck 1992, Lash & Wynne 1992). People come to question the perception that science is the only expert voice. They see that within its own confines, scientific research limits itself as to what it considers worthy of study (often what can be lucratively funded in respect of new technologies and pharmaceuticals). They see that there are other dimensions which science fails to consider which have as much validity as conventional scientific 'facts' (Lash & Wynne 1992). In relation to birth, women see that they need to ask different but precise questions about:

1. whether the technologies used in pregnancy and birth increase or diminish safety
2. how and by whom safety is defined
3. whether the technologies in birth create new complications for the woman and her baby.

Many women see that there are dimensions which conventional or mainstream obstetric science neglects to consider which have decisive impacts on birth and birth outcomes.

An example that has emerged from women's experiences of birth and that has evolved into a reflexive critique with which many midwives are familiar, is that of a routine cardiotocograph (CTG) trace on the woman's admission to a hospital labour ward. The rationale underpinning its routine use is that the technology reduces risk because these readings are accurate. Yet there are no data to support these claims. Studies suggest that admission CTG at best confers no benefit (Impey et al 2003) and at worst leads to increased interventions including, paradoxically, an increase in a woman's exposure to an operative birth (Mires et al 2001). CTG can also affect women's capacities in labour as exemplified in this account:

> I did [feel in control] until I was strapped onto the monitor and then it really changed me. I didn't feel very much in control then but when I was doing all my different positions I was completely in control

> (Edwards 2005)

The awareness (or reflexivity in Beck's terms) of the risks associated with medicalised birth has been a core discourse in the politics of childbirth for the past four decades. Sally Inch's analysis of the 'cascade of intervention' (Inch 1982: 244) captured the concern of women and midwives alike, that in intervening in birth with ever more sophisticated technologies, new hazards and risks were being created. This perspective has been explored by many writers on childbirth since the 1980s.[2]

---

[2] The parameters of this debate are changing however. Davis-Floyd & Dumit (1998) and Pasveer & Akrich (2001) have described how women's relationships to technology are shifting. More fluid and sophisticated technologies give the appearance of increasing women's autonomy, choice and agency. For example, the latest forms of fetal heart monitoring apparently increase women's 'choice'. Surveillance outside the body destroys the argument that technologies are invasive in the conventional sense. But their use reveals an ongoing contest between a discourse promising choice and autonomy and a discourse of control. New technologies can also be invasive in different ways. By controlling the body, they shape women's thinking and expectations in more subtle ways. See Davis-Floyd & Dumit (1998), Gregg (1995), Pasveer & Akrich (2001) and Rothman (1986).

UNMENTIONABLES: THE RISKS THAT ARE NOT COUNTED

Science handles what it thinks it can handle within its model, leaving some risks to be legitimated in its eyes, and some risks and their unseen consequences to be ignored by its experts altogether (Beck 1992). This decision to acknowledge some aspects and to ignore others can increase public disquiet with an impression of 'the two sides talk[ing] past each other' (Beck 1992: 30):

> Social movements raise questions that are not answered by the risk technician at all, and the technicians answer questions which miss the point of what was really asked and what feeds public anxiety

> (Beck 1992)

The decades-long work of campaigning and support organisations like the Association for Improvements in the Maternity Services (AIMS) and the National Childbirth Trust (NCT) are grounded in the effort to overcome these failures of recognition on the part of maternity care providers. Such campaigning organisations have challenged care providers to listen more closely to women's knowledge, experience and anxieties. Women's individual disquiet has been the basis for emerging interpretations of risk and birth which have struggled to be heard and gain recognition alongside the medically dominant versions of risk.

The benefits of obstetric technology and the practices that accompany it have been accepted and made mainstream, often with very little debate. Such mainstreaming draws our attention to the authoritative role that science has played in our lives. Yet the overall costs of technology are profound (Beck 1992, Giddens 1991, Illich 1976, Nelkin 1982) and are often not considered, under-researched, under-reported, minimised or even denied within science. Science, based on the model of laboratory knowledge, measures very 'limited questions'

(Beck 1992: 68) and therefore emerges with limited definitions of safety:

> *so long as risks are not recognised scientifically, **they do not exist** – at least not legally, medically, technologically or socially and thus are not prevented, treated or compensated for*
> (Beck 1992: 71, emphasis in the original)

A good example of this is the use of ultrasound. The side-effects of ultrasound are relatively unknown. There is a presumption of safety; few questions are asked within medical research about its possible adverse impact and it remains an under-researched technology even though it is used routinely. Studies reporting a significant incidence of miscarriage following ultrasound exposure are neither acknowledged nor discussed and questions raised by women remain unanswered (Beech & Robinson 1994).

Lash & Wynne (1992: 4) argue that risk assessment and risk management strategies have become a key part of how science functions. They represent the way that the scientific establishment defends itself against a wider debate because the establishment can argue that it has everything in hand to deal with the risks it creates. As a result, issues that ought to be seriously debated remain unmentionable and uncounted and the opportunity to create further reflexivity is diminished. It is little wonder then that in respect of technologies and birth, it is difficult for us to assess and comprehend the long-term implications. However, women do consistently identify a series of potentially harmful consequences stemming from obstetric practices, especially when obstetric risk categories, rather than women's definitions of safety, become the main organising concept for maternity care. Some women are acutely aware of this:

> *I'm less likely to be subject to unnecessary medical and surgical intervention in my own home so that is the most important aspect of safety that I'm concerned with*
> (Edwards 2005)

Women's ability to make decisions and to act on what they believe is best for them and their babies is limited (Murphy-Lawless 1998a). The morality claims of obstetrics (that women must conform to its strictures if they are to be 'good' mothers), built on top of its truth claims (that it alone knows what really happens in pregnancy and birth) means that obstetrics, in effect, tells women that it is they (the doctors) who are best placed to safeguard the interests of babies. Crucial decisions about babies' lives and deaths are increasingly in the hands of medicine and technology, with little reference to the ethical or quality of life considerations that parents might have (Murphy-Lawless 1998b).

Women's experiences of birth can contest obstetric thinking when they enter the public domain as stories circulated through birth groups, newsletters, maternity consumer panels, or published research. When women reflect on their stories, this process of reflection becomes a tool that helps them challenge obstetrics to consider risk in a radically different way. Women's stories highlight how risk gets defined and by whom and this becomes a political question. This question is positioned alongside the issue of how medical technologies have far higher status than other 'technologies of the body', such as breast stimulation for oxytocic release (Gaskin 1990) or different positions in labour to help the breech birth (Cronk 2005).

Despite the pervasiveness of the risk discourse, women continue to voice their concerns and challenge the authority of obstetric knowledge: they question its logic, assumptions and ethics. Whatever their views about birth, it goes without saying that women are passionately concerned about their own and their babies' safety and that there is no question about abandoning safety as a central concern. What women are saying is clear:

1. that obstetric risk management does not provide real safety in terms of their own and their families' physical, emotional and spiritual health and wellbeing

2. that it creates a whole set of other risks that women feel need to be taken into consideration[3]

3. that it ignores the benefits of a socially supported birth for women and their families.

In the remainder of this chapter, we will draw on the experiences of a group of women (Edwards 2001, 2005) to explore how women's experiences bring them to very different considerations of what constitutes risk in birth. The women's views and experiences were part of extensive fieldwork researching women's decisions and experiences in planning home births in a hospital-based birth culture. This qualitative study involved 30 women who planned home births in Scotland. The women were invited into the study by a letter from community midwives when they booked with NHS community midwifery services for a home birth. The women were aged between 20 and over 40, and came from a variety of economic backgrounds. Most women were white and most were living with partners. There were 13 women who were expecting their first babies and others were expecting second, third and fifth babies. Each woman was interviewed twice before birth and twice after birth. This diverse group of women provided richly reflexive accounts about how women develop different and broader interpretations of risk and safety in childbirth. Their enforced marginalisation, because of their decisions about home birth, enabled them to voice more overtly what many women voice more tentatively.

CHALLENGING THE BASIS OF OBSTETRIC DEFINITIONS OF RISK

Many of these women's views about birth are located against a wealth of experience about the de-emphasising of women's health in modern medicine and the shortcomings of medical certainty:

I would like to challenge some of the things people say. Like for example that the monitoring machine [ultrasound] is completely safe. Nobody knows. You can't say that. They use it and any doctor will say it's safe to use. And they have no right to say that. What they should say is that there's inconclusive evidence, but as far as they know it's okay

(Edwards 2005)

Women question the validity and meaning of applying population-derived data to the individual and to what they judge as complex moral decisions about risk:

I'm not just anybody, you know. I am above average health and fitness probably. My diet is a lot better than most people's. My confidence is probably a lot higher, and my knowledge of birth. And to bunch me in with everybody else without looking at me as an individual, I thought was a very unfair thing. To say that 33% of women need intervention without looking at everything individually, I thought they were being very unfair. But then that's what systems do. You aren't an individual at that level

(Edwards 2005)

Women quickly identify one of the paradoxes of obstetric science: that its own tools, logic and figures do not necessarily support its beliefs. For example, research on place of birth, shows that home birth is as safe as hospital birth for healthy women and babies and that it confers some advantages.[4] They are also aware

---

[3] Risks are both 'real' and 'unreal': real in the sense that many technological hazards are already part of what we must deal with, unreal in the sense that the actual consequences lie in the future and we do not know what shape those consequences may take (Beck 1992: 33–34).

[4] In Britain for example, Campbell & Macfarlane 1994, Chamberlain et al 1997, Davies et al 1996, Ford et al 1991, Northern Regional Perinatal Mortality Survey Coordinating Group 1996, Shearer 1985, Tew 1985, 1998. Elsewhere in Europe and North America research includes that done by Ackermann-Liebrich et al 1996, Anderson & Murphy 1995, Berghs and Spanjaard quoted in Eskes & van Alten 1994, Crotty et al 1990, Durrand 1992, Gaskin 2003, Howe 1988, Johnson & Daviss 2005, Mehl & Peterson 1978, Olsen 1997, Schlenzka 1999, Tyson 1991, Tew & Damstra-Wijmenga 1991, Treffers & Laan 1986, Wayne et al 1987, Wiegers et al 1996, Woodcock et al 1994.

that safety and risk defy simple categorisation and see attempts to portray the hospital setting as one with less risk than the home setting as misleading:

> Everyone kept saying – it's safer to have a baby in hospital, which I thought was disputable, you know. And I thought, there's nothing in life that doesn't come with a risk. Driving to the hospital itself is a risk, and crossing the road is a risk and for them to try and imply that a hospital birth is no risk was misleading.
>
> (Edwards 2005)

From their own experiences, women have concerns about risks similar to those identified by obstetric science. They seek to avoid any obvious risk to their babies during pregnancy and birth. Women also have great concerns about risks which they perceive are less visible to obstetric science, risks that have their origins in the ways births are conventionally managed.

Women describe from their perspectives how, ironically, many aspects of obstetric risk management can create more risk. As we discuss below, the obstetric focus on risk, generalities, routines, time limits, invasive procedures, life at all cost, and its attempts to enforce compliance can decrease safety from their points of view.

THE RISK OF FOCUSING ON RISK

The obstetric focus on risk can be experienced as both pervasive and disempowering, undermining the woman's confidence in her ability to birth her baby. By contrast, the expectation that all will be well unless a complication occurs can be experienced as empowering:

> there seemed to be this big emphasis on prevention – well it's better that you take this drug in case this disaster happens. Or 'It's best you come in hospital 'cos we **don't** want a tragedy', was a quote from the consultant. It was like their focus was very much on fear, which I found completely disempowering. It made me think 'well, maybe I can't deliver a baby.' And I just found myself with a very

weak sort of attitude suddenly. Which was when both my sister and my antenatal teacher suggested an independent midwife. So when I suddenly spoke first to my sister or to my antenatal teacher and then to the independent midwife, the confidence came surging back. It was like, no, this wasn't a figment of my imagination. It is possible to have a home birth.

(Edwards 2001, emphasis in the original)

Many women consider that optimism based on watchfulness, expressed in the midwives' phrase of 'watchful waiting', rather than surveillance generated by pessimism, inspires confidence rather than fear. Within a framework of watchful waiting it follows that it is safer to focus on the likelihood of birth going well than on the risk of birth going wrong. Of course, while dwelling on risk is seen as counterproductive, women want midwives to be ready to respond to complications as necessary.

SUBJECTING INDIVIDUALS TO GENERAL RULES

Wherever women position themselves in relation to birth ideologies they stress the importance of being treated as individuals and the dangers of being subjected to generalised policies and practices. From women's perspectives, one of the riskiest of these general rules is the imposition of obstetric time over a woman's time (Murphy-Lawless 2000). It is difficult to capture in words just how this impacts on the way practitioners respond to women, the pressure women feel under, and the anxiety this causes. There is often a sense of time 'run[ning] on and out' (Adam 1992: 161). This ignores the woman's individual circumstances and leads to obstetric interventions when what women perceive they need, is more time and patient support to give birth. Applying clock time emerges as a strong feature of obstetric thinking. The reality however is that when the institution is under time pressure with its own routines, it fails to carry through its logic. This means that the stated urgency of a situation is met with inaction until the institution has time to act, while ignoring the woman's individual time and bodily knowledge:[5]

> *I wonder if I could have done something about it at home [encouraged labour] if I'd been given a bit more time, and felt that there wasn't such a time issue around it. Which, in fact there wasn't when it turned out, you know. There was a big time lapse in hospital. Cos I hadn't really wanted to do that [have an oxytocin drip] and I suppose looking back on it I think, I should have just said, no, I'm not doing that, I'm just going to let it happen itself, cos it had started. It was just not quick enough*

(Edwards 2005)

INVASIVE PRACTICES AND TECHNOLOGY

While women acknowledge the life-saving attributes of obstetrics and associated procedures, they believe that overuse compromises their own and their babies' safety by potentially imposing physical and emotional pain and harm. So while obstetrics considers birth to be risky and has developed a series of practices to make it 'safe', women not only define these practices as a risk to birth, but talk about the risk of violation:

> *I don't believe that one is less safe in one's own home. On the contrary, I feel that there may be a case to be made that home births*

---

[5] The use of obstetric clock time – 12 hours in the instance of technologies like Active Management of Labour – to manage 'risk' remains largely discredited when used routinely (Schwarz 1990: 56–57, Thornton & Lilford 1994). The application of risk that is the key to Active Management may be inappropriate in any case because the 'majority of infant deaths occur outside the grasp of obstetrical knowledge' (Murphy-Lawless 1998a: 233) and are mainly to be found in material and social poverty and exclusion (Confidential Enquiry into Maternal and Child Health 2004, Murphy-Lawless 2003, Oakley 1992).

> *could be considered safer, if you want to start looking at surgical intervention as a violation of women's bodies*

(Edwards 2005)

Women are not usually afraid of technology in itself. Like those in other studies, they are attached to their babies and families rather than ideologies and have no intention of 'chasing after an ideology' (Lemay 1997: 92). There is a general consensus that prioritising the baby's safety may become inevitable if complications occur:

> *I mean, if the baby's distressed and they say, well, look, you know, we really think we'll have to go in, I'll just go in. I'm not going to risk the baby or myself just because I'm so determined to have a home birth*

(Edwards 2005)

They feel unsafe, however, if they suspect that their other priorities may be ignored, that they might become the unwilling objects of obstetric practices and technology and that their autonomy might be undermined:

> *If there seems to be a problem, I don't want to hold out and have a natural childbirth and a dead baby, or a really unhealthy baby. If the baby's in danger, then of course, do anything. But I suppose it's just if I don't know I'm coming from the same value basis as somebody, then I don't know if they're going to be making decisions on the same basis as I would*

(Edwards 2005)

This points to the importance of women and carers needing to share their values and approaches, and how crucial it is for the carer to listen, to respect the woman's needs and views and to negotiate with these, rather than trying to impose the 'expert' view on women.

LOSS OF AUTONOMY

The rhetoric of choice and control appears to promise women autonomy. However, faced with the powerful obstetric discourse of birth, they are likely to be 'steered' or manipulated

(Kirkham 2004) and as a result they experience a loss of autonomy:

> *I feel like maybe I'm losing control over my responsibility to the baby. I don't feel able to exercise that because I don't really know the situation and I don't know how far to trust the midwives to be doing or understanding what I want*
>
> (Edwards 2005)

Anderson (2004) suggests that supporting women's autonomy is indeed threatening to obstetric ideology. For example, there are now many stories of women expecting breech babies who are planning home births, or attempting to arrange a vaginal breech birth in hospital. In these instances, maternity services have been unable to respond to or facilitate their choices, their autonomy (Anderson 2004, Mahoney 2004). It is the parents themselves who are seen as the risk 'because of their non-compliant behavior' (Viisainen 2000: 810) in wishing to have their babies outside a conventional hospital setting or outside conventional protocols on the handling of breech births. Risk protocols and evidence-based care are too often incompatible with choice, especially if women make decisions that fall outside these protocols and evidence. They prevent midwives being able to talk supportively with women so that women can forge their own decisions (Edwards 2004).

All of the above supports the notion that women in our postmodern but still patriarchal societies are often expected to take responsibility without the means to do so (Benson 2000). Yet as Cronk (2000) suggested, if professionals do not trust or encourage women to retain full responsibility during pregnancy, birth and postnatally, the opportunity for women to develop the abilities, skills and above all the confidence needed to care for their babies and children is undermined. The ability to protect and nurture their children in the context of family life underpins women's views of safe birth. Ignoring this truth presents the ultimate risk that obstetric thinking takes. (Here we use the term 'truth' as found in the work of Badiou (2001), where he defines truth as a form or 'process' of fidelity to a critical event that produces a breakthrough or new way of being for the subject who experiences this event.)

IGNORING RELATIONSHIPS

It is the 'ongoing experience of being a mother to a child' that most radically differentiates the concerns of women from those of obstetrics (Murphy-Lawless 1998a: 47). While the relationships between women and babies and within the family remain invisible in obstetric ideology, protecting and nurturing these relationships is a fundamental priority for mothers. The ongoing decision-making during pregnancy and birth, and how birth is handled, impacts on all intimate relationships. One of the main risks identified by women was the possibility of obstetric ideology and practices undermining these relationships:

> *my responsibility is to form a relationship. It's almost like that the birth is a rite of passage and by the end of it you've been through it together and you're in relationship to the baby. The baby is what comes at the end of the process of giving birth, and I think the more connected I am with the birth, the more connected I am with the baby and maybe my responsibility is to be open to having that connection with the baby*
>
> (Edwards 2005)

Birth here is seen as a rite of passage from which women need to emerge feeling physically and emotionally well in order best to nurture their babies. Yet the strength and importance of that emotional connection is rarely named and tended to by midwives and doctors, especially when they practise in technocratic models of care.

NEGOTIATING RISK AND CHOICE: LIVING WITH UNCERTAINTY

From some women's perspectives, negotiating risk and choice means accepting that uncertainty is inherent to life and that obstetric knowledge and practices cannot eradicate this uncertainty. Indeed, its quest to predict and detect complications has been so unsuccessful (Strong 2000) that all women are considered to be at continual risk or have the potential for risk. This could also be seen as the complete success of obstetric knowledge in that it has managed to imbue every aspect of pregnancy and birth with risk potential. This is of use to its own ambitions to control and monitor every aspect. Women believe that uncertainty exists irrespective of where their babies are born:

> *I suppose for me, I thought, well, you can't guarantee anything in a birth. In a way, you take a risk everytime you enter into it*
>
> (Edwards 2005)

Focusing so strongly on risk alone also undermines the positive potential of pregnancy and birth. This positive potential is not part of obstetric risk discourse, yet Downe's (2004) call for a more positive and subtle focus on salutogenics (a broad sense of wellbeing) rather than risk, is more akin to women's concerns to promote their own, their babies' and their families' health where health means the integration of physical, emotional and spiritual wellbeing.

REDUCING RISK: MAKING CHOICES

Some women believe that the reduction of risk can flow from exerting their autonomy. Both autonomy and safety are enhanced by supportive, competent, confident holistic care during pregnancy and birth from known and trusted midwives who are watchful rather than fearful. But the development of trusting relationships is generally not part of maternity services. Furthermore, the emphasis on obstetric risk management actively prevents the development of alternative views about safety and thus more supportive practices that might enhance this safety are unable to emerge. So for some women, one of the most intractable barriers to their ability to make safe decisions is the way in which obstetric ideology and practices decrease midwives' autonomy and ability to develop alternative birth skills. If women's labours are not completely straightforward, they need

midwives who are able to draw on a range of skills that they know are effective. These are skills that generally work outside or in spite of the constraints of conventional obstetric thinking.

However, while some midwives use birth pools, birth balls and breathing techniques, few have managed to develop the complex of skills and wisdom that enables midwifery to engage with and weave between patterns of birth, culture, and women's emotional responses to birth. The work of building this profound understanding of birth is what distinguishes the kind of midwifery that best supports women to give birth.

Without this extensive range of midwifery skills (that comprise far more than specific techniques) and without the trusting relationships women need, neither women nor midwives can negotiate risk safely or enhance autonomy in labour and birth. Polarisation occurs, with midwives having to work under the shadow of obstetric risk definitions. The heated debates about how breech births should be handled are an example of this polarisation. As Beck (1992: 30) suggests, 'the two sides talk past each other'.

Women are aware of this and worry about the impact of these different and often irreconcilable concerns:

> *if there was a good reason for me going into hospital, I wouldn't trust that it was for a good reason, because I wouldn't know that she [midwife] wasn't just panicking or plotting to get me away*
>
> (Edwards 2005)

Technocratic models prevent midwives developing the experiential and intellectual knowledge, to develop the sort of 'wisdom [that] melts down all the moments of understanding and blends them together to become something more, something deeper and something more open to new understandings' (Smythe 1998: 226). These technocratic models compel mid-wives to stay within the narrow parameters of risk management and apply general rules to individual women, irrespective of women's and midwives' beliefs, values and differences. Without an expanded knowledge base, without a critique of how midwifery struggles within the current power structure, without direct attention to the task of creating more autonomy for their work, midwives cannot enable or respond positively to women's autonomy; they cannot engage with them to enhance safety and respond to risk as labour and birth unfold.

CONCLUSION

Women's narratives underscore a number of crucial issues. Firstly, they are the people most concerned about their own and their babies' wellbeing. Everything they do is about protecting their babies and themselves in order to begin the parenting relationship from the best possible place. In this sense, women who plan home births, elect to have planned caesarean sections, or plan to have unassisted births, share the common desire to be able to minimise harm and maximise wellbeing in order to become self-confident women and mothers.

Secondly, women argue that safety is not an absolute concept and cannot be guaranteed, thus concurring with at least one official position on safety (DH 1993). It seems that safety and autonomy can best be nurtured by increasing women's health and confidence, reducing fear, providing social support, improving holistic midwifery skills, and providing high quality, accessible obstetric services that women and midwives can engage with if and when they need it. There must also be a wider remit to reduce poverty and social exclusion, thereby reducing women's vulnerabilities to poorer physical and mental wellbeing.

Thirdly, women pose a critically important challenge to current birth practices: they are asking whether there are safe, less invasive alternatives to invasive obstetric procedures. They are also asking for skills that reconnect the physiology of the birth process with the emotional needs of women. These are skills that have largely disappeared in a culture that has lost its birth wisdom. The women's definitions of birth suggest the need to draw on wider knowledge pools than the circumscribed knowledge relied on by modern National Health Service maternity care.

We know that poverty, lack of support, and geographical location, for example, continue to impact on the safety of childbearing. But even though this more extensive and grounded vision of midwifery skills remains underdeveloped, a growing body of literature suggests that when midwives are free to respond to women's circumstances, even those most vulnerable to complications remain healthier (Davies 2000, Evans 1987, Rooks 1997).

The way in which risk is currently defined by obstetric science, the risks it ignores, and the way it imposes its risk discourse on women makes it difficult for them to make decisions they believe are right for them if these fall outside the trajectories mapped out for them. Thus, all too often women fear that their integrity will be breached by midwives who are unable to provide the skills they need and in turn, midwives fear that women will want support for situations for which they have been inadequately and inappropriately trained and which lie outside an imposed risk agenda. Yet women's stories suggest that midwifery skills may in some circumstances provide greater safety than technocratic solutions because they achieve the same outcomes but avoid some of the harmful impacts of more invasive technologies. This suggests that changing the balance between midwifery and technocracy would enable the needs of women and midwives to be supported rather than overshadowed by the increasing use of birth technologies.

References

Ackermann-Liebrich U, Voegeli T, Gunter-Witt K et al and Zurich Study Team 1996 Home versus hospital deliveries: follow up study of matched pairs for procedure and outcome. British Medical Journal 313: 1313–1318

Adam B 1992 Time and health implicated: a conceptual critique. In: Frankenberg R (ed) Time, health and medicine. Sage, London, p 153–164

Adam B, Van Loon J 2000 Introduction: repositioning risk: the challenge for social theory. In: Adam B et al (eds) The risk society and beyond: critical issues for social theory. Sage, London

Anderson T 2004 The misleading myth of choice: the continuing oppression of women in childbirth. In: Kirkham M (ed) Informed choice in maternity care. Palgrave Macmillan, Basingstoke, p 257–264

Anderson R, Murphy PA 1995 Outcomes of 11788 planned home births: attended by certified nurse-midwives: a retrospective descriptive study. Journal of Nurse-Midwifery 40: 483–492

Badiou A 2001 Ethics: an essay on the understanding of evil. Verso, London

Bauman Z 1992 Postmodern ethics. Basil Blackwell, Oxford

Bauman Z 1998 Work, consumerism and the new poor. Open University Press, Milton Keynes

Beck U 1992 Risk society: towards a new modernity. Sage, London

Beck-Gernsheim E 2000 Health and responsibility: from social change to technological change and vice versa. In: Adam B et al (eds) The risk society and beyond: critical issues for social theory. Sage, London

Beech BAL, Robinson J 1994 Ultrasound unsound? Association for Improvements in the Maternity Services, c/o 5 Ann's Court, Grove Road, Surbiton, Surrey KT6 4BE. www.aims.org.uk

Benn M 1998 Madonna and child: towards a new politics of motherhood. Jonathan Cape, London

Benson P 2000 Feeling crazy: self-worth and the social character of responsibility. In: Mackenzie C, Stoljar N (eds) Relational autonomy: feminist perspectives on autonomy, agency, and the social self. Oxford University Press, New York and Oxford, p 72–93

Campbell R, Macfarlane A 1994 Where to be born? The debate and the evidence, 2nd edn. National Perinatal Epidemiology Unit, Oxford

Chamberlain G, Wraight A, Crowley P 1997 Home births: the report of the 1994 confidential enquiry by the National Birthday Trust Fund. Parthenon Publishing Group, New York

Confidential Enquiry into Maternal and Child Health 2004 Why mothers die 2000–2002: The Sixth Report on the Confidential Enquiries into Maternal Deaths in the United Kingdom. Royal College of Obstetricians and Gynaecologists, London

Cronk M 2000 The midwife: a professional servant? In: Kirkham M (ed) The midwife–mother relationship. Macmillan, London, p 19–27

Cronk M 2005 Hands off that breech. AIMS Quarterly Journal 17(1): 1–4

Crotty M, Ramsay AT, Smart R et al 1990 Planned home births in Australia 1976–1987. The Medical Journal of Australia 153: 664–671

Davies J 2000 Being with women who are economically without. In: Kirkham M (ed) The midwife–mother relationship, Macmillan, London, p 120–142

Davies J, Hey E, Reid W et al 1996 Prospective regional study of planned home births. British Medical Journal 313: 1302–1306

Davis-Floyd RE 1992 Birth as an American rite of passage. University of California Press, Berkeley, CA

Davis-Floyd RE, Dumit J 1998 Cyborg babies: from techno-sex to techno-tots. Routledge, New York

DH 1993 Changing childbirth: report of the Expert Maternity Group Part 1. HMSO, London

Downe S 2004 Normal childbirth: evidence and debate. Churchill Livingstone, Edinburgh

Downe S, McCormick C, Beech BL 2001 Labour interventions associated with normal birth. British Journal of Midwifery 9(10): 602–606

Durrand AM 1992 The safety of home birth: the Farm study. American Journal of Public Health 82: 450–453

Edwards NP 2001 Women's experiences of planning home births in Scotland: birthing autonomy. PhD thesis, University of Sheffield (unpublished)

Edwards NP 2005 Birthing autonomy: women's experiences of planning home births. Routledge, London

Enkin M 1994 Risk in pregnancy: the reality, the perception and the concept. Birth 21(3): 131–134

Eskes M, van Alten D 1994 Review and assessment of maternity services in the Netherlands. In: Chamberlain G, Patel N (eds) The future of maternity services. RCOG Press, Basingstoke, p 36–46

Evans F 1987 The Newcastle Community Midwifery Care Project: an evaluation report. Newcastle Health Authority, Newcastle upon Tyne

Ford C, Iliffe S, Owen F 1991 Outcome of planned home births in an inner city practice. British Medical Journal 303: 1517–1519

Gaskin IM 1990 Spiritual midwifery. Book Publishing Company, Summertown, Tennessee

Gaskin IM 2003 Ina May's guide to childbirth. Bantam Books, New York

Giddens A 1991 Modernity and identity: Self and identity in the late modern age. Polity Press, London

Glendinning C, Millar J 1992 Women and poverty in Britain: the 1990s. Harvester Wheatsheaf, London

Gregg R 1995 Pregnancy in a high-tech age: paradoxes of choice. New York University Press, New York and London

Howe KA 1988 Home births in south-west Australia. Medical Journal of Australia 149: 296–302

Illich I 1976 Limits to medicine: medical nemesis – the expropriation of health. Marion Boyars, New York

Impey L, Reynolds M, Macquillan K et al 2003 Admission cardiotocography: a randomised controlled trial. Lancet 361: 465–470

Inch S 1982 Birthrights: a parents' guide to modern childbirth. Hutchinson, London

Johnson KC, Daviss B-A 2005 Outcomes of planned home births with certified professional midwives: large prospective study in North America. British Medical Journal 330: 1416

Kirkham M (ed) 2004 Informed choice in maternity care. Palgrave Macmillan, Basingstoke

Lash S, Wynne B 1992 Introduction. In: Beck U Risk society: towards a new modernity. Sage, London

Lemay C 1997 L'accouchement à la maison au Québec: les voix du dedans. MSc thesis, University of Montréal (unpublished)

MacArthur C, Lewis M, Knox G 1991 Health after childbirth. HMSO, London

MacKenzie D 1990 Inventing accuracy: a historical sociology of nuclear missile guidance. MIT Press, Cambridge, MA

Mahoney E 2004 I'll do it my way: a mother's perspective on giving birth to twins. Birth and Beyond 22: 5–8

Martin E 1987 The woman in the body: a cultural analysis of reproduction. Beacon Press, Boston

Mehl LE, Peterson G 1978 Home birth versus hospital birth: comparisons of outcomes of matched populations. In: Ahmed P (ed) Pregnancy, birth and parenting: coping with medical issues. Elsevier-North Holland, New York

Mires G, Williams F, Howie P 2001 Randomised controlled trial of cardiotocography versus Doppler auscultation of fetal heart at admission in labour in low risk obstetric population. British Medical Journal 322: 1457–1460

Murphy-Lawless J 1998a Reading birth and death: a history of obstetric thinking. Cork University Press, Cork

Murphy-Lawless J 1998b Women dying in childbirth: 'Safe motherhood in the international context'. In: Kennedy P, Murphy-Lawless J (eds) Returning birth to women: challenging policies and practices. Centre for Women's Studies, TCD/WERRC, Dublin, p 41–55

Murphy-Lawless J 2000 Midwives, power and women's time in childbirth. Talk at the 1st European Midwifery Congress for Out-of-Hospital Births, 28 September–1 October, Aachen, Germany

Murphy-Lawless J 2003 How will the world be born: the critical importance of indigenous midwifery. Midwives 6(10): 432–436

Nelkin D 1982 Controversy as a political challenge. In: Barnes B, Edge D (eds) Science in context: readings in the sociology of science. Open University Press, Milton Keynes, p 276–281

Northern Regional Perinatal Mortality Survey Coordinating Group 1996 Collaborative survey of perinatal loss in planned and unplanned home births. British Medical Journal 313: 1306–1309

Oakley A 1992 Social support and motherhood. Blackwell, Oxford

O'Connor M 1992 Women and birth – a national study of intentional home births in Ireland. Department of Health, Dublin (unpublished)

Olsen O 1997 Meta-analysis of the safety of home birth. Birth 24(21): 4–13

Pasveer B, Akrich M 2001 Obstetrical trajectories: on training women/bodies for (home) birth. In: DeVries R et al (eds) Birth by design: pregnancy, maternity care, and midwifery in North America and Europe. Routledge, New York, p 229–242

Peterson A 1997 Risk, governance and the new public health. In: Petersen A, Bunton R (eds) Foucault, health and medicine. Routledge, London, p 189–206

Rapp R 1999 Testing women, testing the fetus: the social impact of amniocentesis in America. Routledge, New York

Rooks J 1997 Midwifery and childbirth in America. Temple University Press, Philadelphia, PA

Rothman BK 1986 The tentative pregnancy: prenatal diagnosis and the future of motherhood. Viking Press, New York

Schlenzka PF 1999 Safety of alternative approaches to childbirth. PhD thesis, Stanford University, CA (unpublished)

Schwarz EW 1990 The engineering of childbirth: a new obstetrics programme as reflected in British textbooks, 1960–1980. In: Garcia J, Kilpatrick R, Richards M (eds) The politics of maternity care. Clarendon Paperbacks, Oxford

Shearer JML 1985 Five year survey of risk of booking for a home birth in Essex. British Medical Journal 291: 1478–1480

Smythe E 1998 'Being safe' in childbirth: a hermeneutic interpretation of the narratives of women and practitioners. PhD thesis, Massey University, New Zealand (unpublished)

Strong TH 2000 Expecting trouble: the myth of prenatal care in America. New York University Press, New York

Tew M 1985 Place of birth and perinatal mortality. Journal of the Royal College of General Practitioners 35: 390–394

Tew M 1998 Safer childbirth? A critical history of maternity care, 3rd edn. Free Association Books, London and New York

Tew M, Damstra-Wijmenga SMI 1991 Safest birth attendants: recent Dutch evidence. Midwifery 7: 55–63

Thornton JG, Lilford RJ 1994 Active management of labour: current knowledge and research issues. British Medical Journal 309: 366–368

Treffers PE, Laan R 1986 Regional perinatal mortality and regional hospitalization at delivery in the Netherlands. British Journal of Obstetrics and Gynaecology 93: 690–693

Viisainen K 2000 The moral dangers of home birth: parents' perceptions of risks in home birth in Finland. Sociology of Health and Illness 22(6): 792–814

Wagner M 1994 Pursuing the birth machine: the search for appropriate birth technology. Ace Graphics, Camperdown, NSW

Wayne F, Schramm MA, Barnes DE et al 1987 Neonatal mortality in Missouri home births 1978–84. American Journal of Public Health 77(8): 930–935

Which? Way to Health 1990 Are hospitals the worst place to get well? Which, London

Wiegers T et al 1996 Outcome of planned home and planned hospital births in low risk pregnancies: prospective study in midwifery practices in the Netherlands. British Medical Journal 313: 1309–1313

Woodcock HC, Read AW, Bower C et al 1994 A matched cohort study of planned home and hospital births in Western Australia 1981–1987. Midwifery 10: 125–135

Further Reading

Annandale E 1988 How midwives accomplish natural birth: managing risk and balancing expectations. Social Problems 35(2): 95–110

Bourgeault IL, Benoit C, Davis-Floyd R (eds) 2004 Reconceiving midwifery. McGill-Queen's University Press, Montreal

Devane D, Lalor JG, Daly S et al 2005 Cardiotocography versus intermittent auscultation of fetal heart on admission to labour ward for assessment of fetal wellbeing. (Protocol) The Cochrane Database of Systematic Reviews 2005, Issue 1. Art No: CD005122. DOI: 10.1002/14651858.CD005122

Edwards NP 2004 Why can't women just say no? And does it really matter? In: Kirkham M (ed) Informed choice in maternity care. Palgrave Macmillan, Basingstoke, p 1–29

Garcia J, Kilpatrick R, Richards M (eds) 1990 The politics of maternity care: services for childbearing women in twentieth-century Britain. Clarendon Press, Oxford, p 30–46

Tyson H 1991 Outcomes of 1001 midwife attended home births in Toronto 1983–1988. Birth 18(1): 14–19

Chapter **5**

Risk and Choice in Maternity Care: A View from Action on Pre-eclampsia

Mike Rich

Every woman is unique; every baby is unique; every birth experience is unique. That is why it is so important to give a woman and her partner choice: choice of place of birth; choice of style of care; and choice of professional who is going to accompany them in this unique and special journey

(Cumberlege 2003)

. . . over the next couple of days I had endless visits from doctors and specialists, each offering their own version of what was likely to happen to me. This ranged from being told that if I was a good girl and rested I would be able to go home the next day to being prepared for immediate surgery

(Pre-eclampsia sufferer)

Choice has been, since Changing Childbirth (DH 1993), a hot issue in maternity care. Women are seeking more choice and more information and much of the literature in maternity care in the past decade has been devoted to looking at ways in which extended choice over a woman's pregnancy is given to her. These choices include where to birth, how to birth, interventions that she would prefer not to have, interventions that she would like, pain relief and testing for abnormalities. The choices that face a pregnant woman now far outweigh those that were available to her counterpart 25 years and more ago. On the other hand, with regard to a pregnancy disorder such as pre-eclampsia, risk factors remain relatively similar and a woman's ability to choose may become limited. However, a woman who has suffered from pre-eclampsia can often find herself looking at a range of potential risks and some fundamental choices – one of which is whether to embark on a subsequent pregnancy knowing that she may be putting her own life or the life of her future baby at risk.

> My husband was very traumatized by what happened; we are both very worried about what might happen if I get pregnant again.

> It put me off sex for quite a while. I think that I was scared of getting pregnant again.
>   (Pre-eclampsia sufferer)

Action on Pre-eclampsia is a small single issue maternity charity which was started in 1991 by Isobel Walker and Professor Chris Redman. Isobel had lost a baby due to pre-eclampsia and as a result had set out to find out as much as she could about the disorder. Up until the point that she lost her child, Isobel had not heard of pre-eclampsia. She certainly did not know that it was the most common of the serious complications of pregnancy and that including pregnancy induced hypertension almost 10% of pregnant women were at risk – a figure that was higher in first pregnancies and in women with a variety of other factors.

To her surprise, Isobel found that there were no guides to pre-eclampsia for lay people. What little information that was available to her was limited to a number of medical and academic research papers.

She did not know why she had suffered from pre-eclampsia and at that time she was unaware of the possible risk of having pre-eclampsia again. Without knowledge of those factors and of potential future risk she felt that it was impossible to make choices about any future pregnancies. She set out to find out more and eventually as a medical journalist, and in tandem with Professor Redman, she went on to write a book *Pre-eclampsia: The facts* (Redman & Walker 1992) and founded the charity Action on Pre-eclampsia with the clear aim of educating both women and health professionals as to the prevalence and risks of pre-eclampsia and its complications.

Pre-eclampsia is the most common of the serious pregnancy complications. In its broadest form and including pregnancy induced hypertension it affects approximately 10% of all pregnancies. The risk of pre-eclampsia is greater in first pregnancies where its impact is closer to 20% of pregnancies. Pre-eclampsia and pregnancy induced hypertension affect almost 70 000 pregnancies in the UK every year. Globally, the figures are stark. It is estimated that one woman dies every 6 minutes as a result of pre-eclampsia – mainly due to a lack of antenatal care. The number of babies dying is far, far greater.

Pre-eclampsia is caused by a problem in the placenta as it develops in the first trimester of pregnancy. No one knows for sure what causes pre-eclampsia, although genetic factors are probably involved, since women whose mothers and sisters have suffered pre-eclampsia are more likely to get it themselves. What is known is that pre-eclampsia originates in the placenta. The placenta needs a large and efficient blood supply from the mother to sustain the growing baby. In pre-eclampsia the placenta runs short of blood either because its demands are unusually high – as with twins – or because the arteries in the womb did not enlarge as they should have done when the placenta was being formed in the first half of pregnancy. This shortage of blood has potentially serious consequences for mother and baby.

Signals from the deficient placenta affect the mother's blood vessels, raising her blood pressure and disturbing her kidney function, so that waste products which should be excreted in the urine accumulate in the blood, while valuable blood proteins leak into the urine. As the disease progresses, the mother's liver, lungs, brain and blood clotting system can also be affected. Eclampsia (convulsions), cerebral haemorrhage (stroke), pulmonary oedema (fluid in the lungs), kidney failure, liver damage, and breakdown of the blood clotting system (disseminated intravascular coagulation) are the most dangerous complications – all of them, fortunately, very rare.

Pre-eclampsia continues to be a major cause of poor pregnancy outcome including maternal and fetal mortality and severe obstetric illness. The category 'Hypertensive diseases of pregnancy' remains the second leading cause of direct maternal deaths in the UK (MCHRC 2001a) and pre-eclamptic conditions (severe pre-eclampsia, HELLP syndrome, eclampsia) represent 1 in 3 cases of severe obstetric morbidity (Waterstone et al 2001).

> *After suffering from HELLP syndrome I acted on my consultant's advice and terminated my next pregnancy at seven weeks*
>
> (Pre-eclampsia sufferer)

For the baby, hypertension and/or proteinuria is the leading single identifiable risk factor in pregnancy associated with stillbirth (1 in 5 stillbirths in otherwise viable babies), about 7% of which are directly caused by pre-eclampsia (MCHRC 1999, 2001b). Pre-eclampsia is also associated with fetal growth restriction, low birth weight, preterm delivery, small for gestational age (SGA) infants and respiratory distress syndrome (Altman et al 2002).

Most of the deaths due to pre-eclampsia have been associated with substandard care and with two main areas within primary care. One is the failure to identify and act on known risk factors at booking and the second is the failure to recognise and act appropriately on signs and symptoms from 20 weeks' gestation. In 80% of maternal deaths and 65% of fetal deaths, the woman and baby received 'major substandard' care: in other words, care that contributed significantly to the death, and where different management would reasonably have been expected to alter the outcome (MCHRC 1999, 2001a,b).

> *I struggled to come to terms with the loss of my baby and the fear that I may never be able to have another child.*
>
> (Pre-eclampsia sufferer)

Pre-eclampsia is serious. It is serious for the baby and it is serious for the mother. In spite of this, for the majority of women who contact our charity often the first time they had heard of pre-eclampsia was when they were being admitted into hospital for observation, an induced birth or an emergency caesarean. They were unaware of the risk and now much choice

is being taken away by a potential clinical emergency.

In 2004 Action on Pre-eclampsia published a guideline for the identification of risk and the management of pre-eclampsia within the community setting (Milne et al 2005).

THE PRE-ECLAMPSIA COMMUNITY GUIDELINE (PRECOG)

It is a widely accepted policy that maternity service users – the pregnant women themselves – have a full and equal right to determine and be involved in their antenatal care and on that basis, the mother's full involvement in the antenatal care plan outlined in the PRECOG guideline has been assumed.

Women can only do this if they are given the opportunity to have an understanding of the relevance of the process to themselves and their babies from the first contact with the healthcare professional. Information leaflets for pregnant women are available as part of the PRECOG package. Providers have an obligation to make appropriate information available to women in these circumstances.

An individual and flexible antenatal care plan can then be developed by all concerned which takes fully into account the emotional needs and cultural issues of the pregnant woman, her individual likelihood of developing pre-eclampsia and any specialist input to care that has been identified. In this way a pregnant woman can be reassured that she has the best possible antenatal care plan for her and her baby, enabling her to have the confidence to enjoy her pregnancy, whatever her likelihood of developing pre-eclampsia.

While the development of pre-eclampsia will undoubtedly have an impact on the breadth of choices that a woman has, it is important that she has control over both the level of information she has and the choices that are available within her particular situation. Some writers on choice have criticised what choice is available for women as the ability of choosing options from a limited menu rather than a 'full' ability to choose. Undoubtedly, this criticism could be levelled at the choice that can become available to a woman who has developed pre-eclampsia. The question that we find ourselves asking is – what constitutes 'full' choice and is it realistic in a situation in which a woman has particular clinical needs?

WHAT ARE THE RISKS OF PRE-ECLAMPSIA AND WHAT PART CAN A WOMAN PLAY IN MITIGATING THEM OR CONSIDERING HER CHOICES?

Age is a significant factor. As we are moving towards a period in which a larger number of women are leaving their pregnancies until later on in life, and that those later pregnancies are at increased risk of complication, it is a key area in which a woman can view herself as having a choice – indeed, choice is often the key to why women are having their children later on in life.

In a systematic review of evidence papers carried out by Duckitt & Harrington (2005) on behalf of Action on Pre-eclampsia women aged over 40 were found to be approaching twice the risk of developing pre-eclampsia. While all except one of the studies failed to control or address differences at baseline (particularly pre-existing chronic disease such as hypertension or diabetes) women aged over 40 had almost twice the risk whether or not they were primiparous or multiparous. It is also not clear that the age of 40 is an ideal cutoff when looking at risk – although from a clinical point of view it is practical – as some nationwide US data suggest that the risk of pre-eclampsia increases by 30% for every additional year of age past 34 (Saftlas et al 1990). While it has often been thought that pre-eclampsia was more prevalent among teenagers, Duckitt & Harrington's systematic review did not suggest that young maternal age affected the risk of developing pre-eclampsia whichever cutoff age was used.

Being a first-time mother impacts considerably on the risk of developing pre-eclampsia, although the issue of choice in this case is a moot one.

Nulliparous women are almost three times more likely to get pre-eclampsia as multiparous ones and women with pre-eclampsia are almost twice as likely to be nulliparous as women without pre-eclampsia.

For a charity such as Action on Pre-eclampsia the question that is most asked of us is 'Will I get it again?' Unfortunately, the answer to the question is 'possibly'. Women who have pre-eclampsia in a first pregnancy have seven times the risk of pre-eclampsia in a second pregnancy. Women with pre-eclampsia in their second pregnancy are also more than seven times more likely to have a history of pre-eclampsia in their first pregnancy than women in their second pregnancy who do not develop pre-eclampsia. With regard to the question of choice this is where the charity does most of its work. Will I get it again, will it affect me in the same way, what are the risks to my baby, what are the risks to me, and can anything be done to ameliorate the risks? These are the everyday questions that are asked on the Action on Pre-eclampsia Helpline.

Women who have suffered from pre-eclampsia are exceptionally concerned about the possible risks of developing pre-eclampsia again and I have spoken to many women who have decided not to pursue a subsequent pregnancy and to those who have put off a subsequent pregnancy for 5–10 years after their first experience of pre-eclampsia.

A FAMILY HISTORY OF PRE-ECLAMPSIA

For those women who have had a mother or sister who has developed pre-eclampsia, their risk of developing it themselves is almost tripled and there is even a small risk if their mother-in-law has suffered from pre-eclampsia. For health professionals advising women on risks in their pregnancy, the taking of a thorough history at the booking appointment is an important task. While the risk factors that I have mentioned have not been combined to give an idea of risk for a woman with multiple risk factors, the woman who presents at booking as a primiparous woman whose sister has suffered from severe pre-eclampsia in the past 10 years is clearly significantly more at risk from developing the disorder herself, and should be given full information as to the possible impact of the disorder on her pregnancy and how it will affect the choices that she has.

Multiple pregnancy is a key factor in the development of pre-eclampsia. A woman who is pregnant with twins has nearly triple the risk of developing pre-eclampsia while a woman who is pregnant with a triplet pregnancy nearly triples her risk of pre-eclampsia in comparison to a twin pregnancy. At a time when more people are delaying starting their families until later and the increase in the opportunities for assisted reproduction, more women are having twin and triplet pregnancies at a later age. It is clear that these women need to be counselled as to their increased risks of pre-eclampsia which could compromise their pregnancy. Pre-conception counselling in this case should be aimed at helping the woman make realistic choices based upon a full knowledge of the complications that may come with an assisted later pregnancy.

PRE-EXISTING MEDICAL CONDITIONS

INSULIN DEPENDENT DIABETES

The likelihood of pre-eclampsia nearly quadruples if diabetes is present before pregnancy and it is important that women who have diabetes are counselled as to their risk of developing pre-eclampsia.

PRE-EXISTING HYPERTENSION

In a population based nested case-control study, Davies et al found that the prevalence of chronic hypertension was higher in women who developed pre-eclampsia than women who did not. McCowan et al (1996) compared outcomes in 129 women with chronic hypertension who did not develop superimposed pre-eclampsia with 26 women with chronic hypertension who did. Those with superimposed pre-eclampsia had significantly higher rates of perinatal morbid-

ity, small for gestational age infants and delivery before 32 weeks. A diastolic blood pressure before 20 weeks of either greater than or equal to 110 mmHg (5.2, 1.5 to 17.2) or greater than or equal to 100 mmHg (3.2, 1.0 to 7.8) (Duckitt & Harrington 2005) is most predictive in the development of superimposed pre-eclampsia.

RENAL DISEASE

Davies et al also found that the prevalence of renal disease was higher in women who developed pre-eclampsia compared with those who did not (5.3% v. 1.8%).

OTHER FACTORS

TIME BETWEEN PREGNANCIES

In a Norwegian population study Skjaerven et al (2002) studied 551 478 women who had two or more singleton deliveries and 209 423 women who had three or more singleton deliveries. The association between risk of pre-eclampsia and interval was more significant than the association between risk and change of partner. The risk in a second or third pregnancy was directly related to the time elapsed since the previous delivery. When the interval was 10 years or more the risk of pre-eclampsia was about the same as that in nulliparous women. After adjustment for the presence or absence of a change of partner, maternal age, and year of delivery, the probability of pre-eclampsia was increased by 1.12 for each year increase in the interval. A cross-sectional study from Uruguay found that women with more than 59 months between pregnancies had significantly increased risks of pre-eclampsia compared with women with intervals of 18–23 months. A Danish cohort study found that a long interval between pregnancies was associated with a significantly higher risk of pre-eclampsia in a second pregnancy when pre-eclampsia had not been present in the first pregnancy and paternity had not changed.

For some time it has been thought that a change of partner was likely to increase the risk of pre-eclampsia. This has led to many incidences in which women have been asked very awkward questions about paternity – it is now thought that rather than the increased risk being from a change of partner it is more likely associated with the gap between pregnancies as outlined above, with women who change partners often more likely to leave a greater gap between pregnancies than women who stay with the same partner.

BODY MASS INDEX

Although the studies that looked at body mass index before pregnancy all used different ranges, they all showed effects in the same direction, suggesting an overall doubling of risk of pre-eclampsia with a raised body mass index. One cohort study showed that women with a body mass index >35 before pregnancy had over four times the risk of pre-eclampsia compared with women with a pre-pregnancy body mass index of 19–27 (Bianco et al 1998). A combination of all studies that looked at raised compared with normal body mass index at booking found that the risk of pre-eclampsia is increased by 50% (Sibai et al 1997). Notably, a body mass index of >35 at booking doubles the pre-eclampsia risk. Confounding factors can affect the relation between body mass index and pre-eclampsia as women with raised body mass index may be older and more at risk of chronic hypertension. However, published odds ratios that have been adjusted to take some of these factors into account still suggest an increased risk with a raised body mass index. A study comparing low and normal body mass index at booking found that the risk of pre-eclampsia was significantly reduced with a body mass index. It is clear that a reduction in a woman's body mass index would have an impact on her risk of pre-eclampsia and it has been thought for some time by some doctors that obese women should be counselled as to the extra risks that are involved in a pregnancy due to obesity.

BLOOD PRESSURE AT BOOKING

Reiss et al (1987) matched 30 women with pre-eclampsia for age, race and parity with

Table 5.1 Risk factors for pre-eclampsia

Factor	Unadjusted relative risk	(95% CI)
Previous pre-eclampsia	7.19	5.85–8.83
Antiphospholipid antibodies	9.72	4.34–21.75
Diabetes	3.56	2.54–4.99
Family history	2.90	1.70–4.93
Multiple pregnancy (twins)	2.93	2.04–4.21
First pregnancy	2.91	1.28–6.61
Age 40 or more (multip)	1.96	1.34–2.87
Age 40 or more (primip)	1.68	1.23–2.87
BMI raised at booking	1.55	1.28–1.88
Diastolic blood pressure at booking	1.38	1.01–1.87

Meta-analysis of factors measured in early pregnancy that increase the likelihood of pre-eclampsia (Duckitt & Harrington 2005). BMI, body mass index.

normotensive control women. Both systolic and diastolic blood pressures were significantly higher in the first trimester for women who later developed pre-eclampsia. Sibai et al (1995) found that higher systolic and diastolic blood pressures at the first visit were associated with an increased incidence of pre-eclampsia.

Clearly there is a range of risk factors for pre-eclampsia of which women should be made aware. An increased chance of pre-eclampsia may have an impact on the ability of a woman to have a home birth as opposed to a hospital birth. It may mean that she needs to make a birth plan that is more 'flexible' than she would otherwise like. It may mean an increased amount of medical intervention.

What is clear from the women that Action on Pre-eclampsia works with is that while there is an acceptance that the risks of developing pre-eclampsia may have a significant impact on their realistic choices, it is more important that the risks are clearly explained to them in order that they can understand and still make what choices are available to them.

HOW ARE WOMEN AFFECTED BY PRE-ECLAMPSIA AND WHAT DIFFERENCE DOES IT MAKE TO THEIR LIVES AND FUTURE CHOICES?

Action on Pre-eclampsia has been operating a helpline for over 10 years, supporting women and their families when there has been a diagnosis of pre-eclampsia. We have collected a vast amount of anecdotal evidence which suggests that for a large percentage of women their experience of pre-eclampsia has had a considerable impact on not only their experience of and feelings about their pre-eclamptic pregnancy but also their attitudes to future pregnancies.

HOW DO WOMEN FEEL AFTER BEING AFFECTED BY PRE-ECLAMPSIA?

Action on Pre-eclampsia has been collecting anecdotal information from women for over 10 years, however in 2004/5 we decided to carry out a survey of our membership to find out how women had been affected and, importantly, to find out how their experience had affected them emotionally.

The organisation has a membership of approximately 900 individuals all of whom pay an annual subscription for which they receive a comprehensive information pack, newsletters and email updates.

THE MEMBERSHIP SURVEY

The membership survey had 91 questions in total, with separate sections for up to six pregnancies for each respondent. The questions covered:

- Risk factors for pre-eclampsia
- Obstetric history
- Neonatal history
- Physical health after pre-eclampsia
- Emotional health after pre-eclampsia
- Evaluation of ante- and postnatal care and
- Evaluation of the services that we offer them at Action on Pre-eclampsia.

The initial response rate was just under 20%, which was slightly disappointing; however, we recognised that this may have been due to the number and types of question that were asked and the fact that it is sometimes difficult for women who have had poor pregnancy experiences to discuss them subsequently. Since the initial questionnaire was distributed, we have carried out further distributions and now hope to have a subsequent analysis which will account for approximately 40% of our membership. The figures presented here are, however, based on the initial analysis.

It is important to state that the data that we have were taken from our membership who are a self-selected sample, all of whom had all contacted and subsequently joined the charity after a pregnancy complicated by pre-eclampsia. It is clear that the experiences that they have outlined come from the more acute end of the spectrum and as such represent those women who have been seriously rather than mildly affected.

The analysis of the whole survey is well beyond the scope of this chapter. Instead we have concentrated on the information that we gathered from the first pregnancy (beyond 20 weeks) of each respondent which gives a snapshot image of our membership.

RISK FACTORS FOR PRE-ECLAMPSIA

Analysis of the risk factors for pre-eclampsia showed that out of the 172 respondents:

- 94% experienced pre-eclampsia in their first pregnancy
- 33% had a mother or a sister affected by pre-eclampsia (a couple also talked about having mothers-in-law affected)
- 7% had had twin pregnancies
- 1% had pre-existing kidney problems or diabetes mellitus
- 1% suffered from antiphospholipid syndrome

DIAGNOSIS

93% of the cases of pre-eclampsia were diagnosed before labour. The earliest diagnosis was at 19 weeks, in a woman who suffered from chronic hypertension; as pre-eclampsia can only be clinically diagnosed from 20 weeks' gestation, in this case there may have been an issue with agreed dates of conception. The latest was at 42 weeks.

- 93% pre-labour
- 5% during labour
- 2% after delivery
- 41% noticed the symptoms themselves
- 11% reported that their symptoms were not acted upon

SYMPTOMS

With regard to information that had been supplied to women it is interesting to note that almost half of the women noticed symptoms themselves in spite of the key symptoms of pre-eclampsia – high blood pressure and protein in the urine – being exceptionally difficult to identify outside an antenatal appointment.

- 92% had hypertension
- 90% had proteinuria
- 87% were oedematous
- 53% suffered from headaches
- 40% reported visual disturbances
- 37% had epigastric pain
- 36% experienced reduced fetal movement

The other most commonly mentioned symptom was nausea.

OBSTETRIC OUTCOMES

Of these women:

- 17% developed eclampsia
- 27% suffered from HELLP syndrome
- 11% had placental abruptions while overall
- 38% were admitted to intensive care
- there was 1 maternal death

NEONATAL OUTCOMES

Of the 172 pregnancies sampled, 179 babies were born; of these:

- 17% were stillborn

- 83% were live births; however of these 149 live births, 34 babies (23%) subsequently died, typically in the first week
- 63% of all the babies born were admitted to neonatal intensive care unit

EMOTIONAL HEALTH AFTER PRE-ECLAMPSIA

Emotional health is one of the key issues which often affects a woman's decision to embark on a subsequent pregnancy or not. As such we were particularly interested in women's emotional health after pregnancies affected by pre-eclampsia. Some of the figures strengthened the observations of the people who worked on our helpline. Of the sample, 14% were diagnosed with postnatal depression including some women (and men) who went on to be diagnosed with post-traumatic stress disorder. Almost half of the sample reported suffering from a range of emotional problems (43%) while 40% reported that they had had relationship difficulties as a result of them suffering from pre-eclampsia although this figure has not been broken down into those women whose baby had survived against those whose baby had died. A massive 19% of the women surveyed reported that they had decided not to go on with any subsequent pregnancy as they were concerned about the risk of developing pre-eclampsia again.

- 14% of the sample were diagnosed with postnatal depression
- 43% reported suffering from emotional problems
- 40% had relationship difficulties
- 19% decided against any further pregnancies

Although we asked the respondents to give details of the emotional problems they had suffered from, they did not all specify these. Those who did enlarge on the question mentioned post-traumatic stress disorder, guilt and anxiety. Many of the women who answered the question suffered from long-term clinical depression and many of those who had suffered bereavement found it difficult to come to terms with this.

I felt very guilty and very angry for a long time. I worried that perhaps it was my fault that I had become so ill and my baby had suffered.

(Pre-eclampsia sufferer)

Feelings of guilt were a constant theme and of particular concern to Action on Pre-eclampsia. Pre-eclampsia is a pathological condition that individuals can do little about. We have discussed some of the areas that make you more prone to developing pre-eclampsia and that a woman could conceivably have some impact on (obesity and age). However, for most women the risk factors are such that they are effectively out of the hands of the individual. Yet the question is still asked: Was it something I did? What can I do in my next pregnancy that will make me less likely to develop pre-eclampsia?

In this section of the survey we asked the respondents to specify the emotional problems that they were having and the kind of support that they received. Not everyone filled in this section, but of those who did some mentioned post-traumatic shock disorder, while others discussed guilt and anxiety; many suffered from long-term depression, and bereavement was also a theme.

The respondents found support in many different and some unusual places. However, an overwhelming number indicated that their general practitioners (GPs), midwives and health visitors had played a significant role in helping them come to terms with the outcomes of their pregnancies.

EVALUATION OF ANTENATAL AND POSTNATAL CARE

- 58% of the sample were happy with their antenatal care
- 33% were happy with their postnatal care
- only 6% made an official complaint about their care
- 1 legal action resulted

Many of the women who contact our charity after a pregnancy affected by pre-eclampsia are anxious to understand exactly what had happened to them and why.

It was very reassuring to be offered both an explanation of what had occurred and a plan of action for my next pregnancy.

(Pre-eclampsia sufferer)

INFORMATION RECEIVED AFTER PREGNANCY AFFECTED BY PRE-ECLAMPSIA

The membership survey found that after being discharged from hospital only:

- 16% of the sample had been given a written explanation about their experience of pre-eclampsia
- 35% received a verbal explanation, however many of them noted that this was usually given to them when they were either too traumatised by what had happened or too eager to get home to really take in what was being said to them

As a charity one of our most important objectives is to provide information and support for women and their families after a pregnancy affected by pre-eclampsia. The majority of the women we speak to are often confused about what has happened to them and their pregnancies. It is clear from the figures above that information given postpartum is either not sufficient or happens at a time when the women are not in a position to take on board what is being told to them.

So what of risk and choice for the woman at risk of pre-eclampsia? For Action on Pre-eclampsia it is vitally important that all women who are potentially at risk should have a clear understanding of the signs and symptoms of the disorder and the impact that it may have on their pregnancy. For women at lower risk, it is clear that the choices available to them should be in line with those available to all low risk pregnant women. For those at high risk, the options are not quite so clear. The development of pre-eclampsia is difficult to predict, can progress to a crisis very quickly and can prove fatal to both mother and baby. In these circumstances, choice will be of necessity limited. It may be necessary to bring a woman who has been diagnosed with pre-eclampsia into hospital even though, at that

Case Study
It is Better that You Don't Know

This would have been a cause for rejoicing had I not still felt the bump-bump of anxiety, and the ever-present headache. A brisk lady doctor stood at the foot of the bed and pronounced me fit to go. 'Is there anything I should look out for?' I asked. She avoided my eyes, looking only at my notes, which she held with both hands, tapping her foot on the lino. 'Oh, if your headache gets worse, see your GP', she said in an offhand manner. 'Anything else I

should know?' I persisted. 'Oh, if you get chest pain go and see your doctor', 'Chest pain?' I asked, 'What kind of chest pain?' Suddenly she looked at me for the first time. 'It is better that you do not know', she said. 'I disagree', I heard my voice quiet and determined. I would meet what she had to tell me. I was ready for the bad news.

'Look!' she said, 'There are some things it is better that you do not know!'

---

point, she feels well. It may be necessary to induce the birth, it may be necessary to perform a caesarean section, in an emergency or elective. While choice may be limited and the woman may be offered an exceptionally limited 'menu', the important element of this situation is that the woman should be made fully aware of the risks involved and the clinical options that are open to both her and her doctors.

It is my opinion that a woman who is at high risk of developing pre-eclampsia needs early guidance on the possible outcomes of her pregnancy. While she may well go to term and deliver her baby in a 'normal' way with choices over interventions and the birth process she must also be aware of the other potential outcomes – what might happen if there is a need for induction, what might happen if there is a need for a caesarean. While it may feel that this approach may prematurely limit a woman's choices, the reality is that it may well empower in a situation that is not easily predicted. While many women have told us that knowing what might happen can cause anxiety, they feel that this is preferable to not knowing and then being faced with a clinical situation that they do not understand and that they have no control over whatsoever.

References

Altman D, Carroli G, Duley L et al 2002 Do women with pre-eclampsia, and their babies, benefit from magnesium sulphate? The Magpie Trial: a randomised placebo-controlled trial. Lancet 359: 1877–1890

Bianco AT, Smilen SW, Davi Y et al 1998 Pregnancy outcome and weight gain recommendations for the morbidly obese woman. Obstetrics and Gynecology 91: 97–102

Cumberlege (Baroness) 2003 House of Lords Debate, 15 January 2003, cols 267–268

Davies AM, Czaczkes JW, Sadovsky E et al 1970 Toxemia of pregnancy in Jerusalem I. Epidemiological studies of a total community. Israel Journal of Medical Sciences 6: 253–266

DH 1993 Changing Childbirth (The report of the Expert Maternity Group). HMSO, London

Duckitt K, Harrington D 2005 Risk factors for pre-eclampsia at antenatal booking: systematic review of controlled studies. British Medical Journal 330: 565–572

McCowan LM, Buist RG, North RA et al 1996 Perinatal morbidity in chronic hypertension. British Journal of Obstetrics and Gynaecology 103: 123–129

MCHRC (Maternal and Child Health Research Consortium) 1999 Confidential Enquiries into Stillbirths and Deaths in Infancy. 6th report. MCHRC, London,

MCHRC (Maternal and Child Health Research Consortium) 2001a Confidential enquiries into maternal deaths. MCHRC, London

MCHRC (Maternal and Child Health Research Consortium) 2001b Confidential Enquiries into Stillbirths and Deaths in Infancy. 8th report. MCHRC, London

Milne F, Redman C, Walker J et al 2005 The pre-eclampsia community guideline (PRECOG): how to screen for and detect onset of pre-eclampsia in the community. British Medical Journal 330: 576–580

Redman C, Walker I 1992 Pre-eclampsia: The facts – the hidden threat to pregnancy. Oxford Medical Publications, Oxford

Reiss RE, O'Shaughnessy RW, Quilligan TJ et al 1987 Retrospective comparison of blood pressure course during preeclamptic and matched control pregnancies. American Journal of Obstetrics and Gynecology 156: 894–898

Saftlas AF, Olson DR, Franks AL et al 1990 Epidemiology of pre-eclampsia and eclampsia in the United States, 1979–1986. American Journal of Obstetrics and Gynecology 163: 460–465

Sibai BM, Gordon T, Thom E et al 1995 Risk factors for preeclampsia in healthy nulliparous women: a prospective multicenter study. American Journal of Obstetrics and Gynecology 172: 642–648

Sibai BM, Ewell M, Levine RJ et al 1997 Risk factors associated with preeclampsia in healthy nulliparous women. The Calcium for Pre-eclampsia Prevention Study Group. American Journal of Obstetrics and Gynecology 177: 1003–1010

Skjaerven R, Wilcox AJ, Lie RT 2002 The interval between pregnancies and the risk of preeclampsia. New England Journal of Medicine 346: 33–38

Waterstone M, Bewley S, Wolfe C et al 2001 Incidence and predictors of severe obstetric morbidity: case-control study. Commentary: Obstetric morbidity data and the need to evaluate thromboembolic disease. British Medical Journal 322: 1089–1094

Chapter **6**

Risk and Choice: a View From an Inner City Teaching Hospital in the UK

Sinead McNally

BACKGROUND TO THE DEVELOPMENT OF RISK MANAGEMENT IN THE UNIT

This chapter addresses risk management and incident reporting in a large inner city teaching hospital which has approximately 6000 births per annum. Clinical Governance is best described in terms of continuous quality improvement in practice. It involves both a corporate and individual approach to 'doing anything and everything required to maximise quality' (Lilley 1999: 109). But the challenge of Clinical Governance from the outset was to understand and implement strategies that could be employed to demonstrate a true commitment to changing and improving practice. One strategy was the application of risk management principles from industry to the National Health Service (NHS) (DH 2000).

Risk management is focusing less on avoiding or mitigating claims and is now described more in terms of being a tool for improving practice. Risk management thus can be described as one of the pillars, routes or branches of Clinical Governance (Chambers & Wakley 2000).

Across Scotland in many maternity units risk management is only one part of a particular person's role (SPCERH 2004). This means that a midwife or other member of the maternity team split their duties between clinical care and risk management. In 2000 the Simpson Centre for Reproductive Health (SCRH) demonstrated a corporate commitment by appointing a full-time Clinical Risk Coordinator for Reproductive Health. Cooper (2000) suggested that any unit with more than 4500 births per annum should have a full-time Risk Coordinator. In 2000 the SCRH had in excess of 5000 births per year. On appointment, the Clinical Risk Coordinator undertook benchmarking visits to other UK maternity units of a similar size. The strengths and weaknesses of several approaches to incident reporting and risk management in general were collated. Incident reporting is one of the key activities of risk management. The analysis of the reported events and dissemination of 'lessons learnt' to both management and all members of the multidisciplinary team involved in maternity care became a goal of the SCRH in 2000. The approach adopted was to create and foster a culture where risk management was not a person or the name of a department but instead risk management activities were undertaken by all managers and practitioners. As befits a large teaching hospital, there were many 'meetings' in the SCRH where 'cases' were discussed.

There were weekly Perinatal Meetings where selected babies who were admitted to the Neonatal Unit were discussed. A review of antenatal, intrapartum and postnatal care and decision-making was presented. Following this the members of the multidisciplinary team participated in discussion, often comparing the quality of the management with current evidence.

At the monthly Perinatal Mortality meeting the cases of women who had recently suffered a perinatal loss were presented in a similar manner. At this meeting there was the advantage of input from the pathology department and the findings of the postmortem were presented and discussed.

Monthly Cardiotocograph (CTG) Meetings were held where labour and birth records were reviewed, the fetal heart traces scrutinised and the decision-making processes in labour were discussed.

The anaesthetic staff held monthly meetings to discuss cases of interest or cases involving adverse outcomes or cases of severe maternal morbidity.

In 2000–01 these meetings were seen largely as the preserve of the medical staff. Records of attendance, the issues discussed and dissemination of 'lessons learnt' were not fed back to most of the unit staff. An educational drive was undertaken to encourage more staff (particularly theatre and midwifery staff) to attend and participate in discussions regarding decision-making and outcomes in maternity and neonatal care.

The attendance rose from approximately 20 to 70 by 2004 and the attendance records have continued to show a significant rise in the attendance by midwives, theatre staff, and midwifery and medical students. Midwives in particular were encouraged and supported in joining in these often volatile and sometimes confrontational gatherings. (Where a poor outcome is known prior to the presentation there is a temptation on the part of the audience to finger point, and an atmosphere of negativity and censure rather than true multidisciplinary learning may ensue.)

These joint meetings were in keeping with the recommendation following the observation in the Confidential Enquiries into Maternal and Child Health (CEMACH) report that 'midwives appeared to have missed the opportunity to question the decisions made by other professionals and advocate for the women in their care' (CEMACH 2004). To achieve this, midwives must have a sound knowledge base and be able to have the confidence to voice their concerns. A non-judgmental learning approach is now encouraged in all case discussions in the SCRH.

'Risk management feedback sessions' introduced staff to the background and functions of the Clinical Negligence Scheme for Trusts (CNST) in England and the Clinical Negligence and Other Risk Indemnity Schemes (CNORIS) in Scotland. The recommendations from national and international reports were also presented on a regular basis (CESDI 1999, CEMD 1999, CEMACH 2004, DH 2000).

INCIDENT REPORTING AS A TOOL FOR LEARNING AND IMPROVING PRACTICE

At a busy tertiary unit such as the SCRH the role of the Clinical Risk Coordinator at the outset was to raise awareness of incident reporting and lessons that could be learned from practice.

A vision for risk management in five steps was disseminated to staff:

1. minimise the risk of patients (i.e. mothers and babies) coming to harm
2. foster a safe environment for staff and visitors
3. maintain a good reputation of the service
4. promote a just and fair culture where all members of the multidisciplinary team take responsibility for their actions, report incidents and learn from incident feedback sessions
5. match compliance with local, national and international standards where appropriate

The terminology of risk management is continuously changing. What was referred to as 'adverse outcomes' and 'near miss' (DH 2000) have now been replaced with 'patient safety incident' and 'severe morbidity' (NPSA 2004). The term 'no blame culture' had been recommended by the expert group involved in compiling the report on risk management in the NHS (DH 2000) to encourage an open approach to incident reporting. It has many supporters (Green 2001, Richardson 2002) but the term may also suggest a 'laissez faire' approach to reducing risk. The National Patient Safety Agency (2004) has suggested that a 'no blame culture' is neither desirable nor feasible. After a thorough investigation, disciplinary action may be the action required in *rare* cases (Taylor-Adams & Vincent 2004). Staff in the maternity unit welcomed and approved of a culture of no blame and a 'no blame statement' was added to the incident form. This addition is no longer possible as an electronic incident form has been introduced but staff are reminded that the SCRH continues to foster a no unjustified blame culture on the Risk Management web page of the hospital.

The emphasis in risk management circles has begun to shift rapidly from a 'no blame' culture to a culture of safety, a culture of accountability and a culture of learning (Currie et al 2004, Simpson 2000).

A shift also occurred in that the aim of risk management has moved away from reducing litigation as a major outcome to one where all staff buy into the idea/concept that 'risk management' is about improving care. Litigation commonly arises in the context of poor quality care, and risk management should reduce outcomes that lead to claims, although this is not its sole or primary purpose. 'Risk management is as much about learning from claims as it is about mitigating claims' (RCOG 2005: 2).

'REAL–TIME' INCIDENT REPORTING ON THE LABOUR SUITE

On appointment the Clinical Risk Coordinator explored strategies to improve staff awareness of the benefit of incident reporting. One successful strategy was the introduction of Real-Time incident reporting on the labour suite. This was designed to overcome some of the barriers to incident reporting and risk management such as lack of feedback and the lack of appreciation of a systems approach to safety events (Cozens-Firth et al 2004, Kingston et al 2004, Reason 2001).

The idea of a daily, multidisciplinary forum to discuss the incidents reported in the previous 24 hours was introduced to the labour suite in October 2001 by a visiting obstetrician from the Liverpool Women's Hospital. In December 2001 'Real Time' began on the labour suite. This term is used mainly in aviation, the nuclear industry and the space programme. It refers to the speed at which feedback is available and 'the timeliness of the feedback itself' (Quinn 2003).

Feedback from Real Time is also presented at the Labour Suite Management Committee, which has two lay members in the group. Their views on risk-reducing recommendations and the issue of women's choice are addressed later in the chapter.

Incident reporting had been a feature on the labour suite since 1998, when six or seven incidents were reported a month. At that stage the Clinical Manager for the labour suite along with obstetric and anaesthetic staff reviewed the maternal records.

The labour suite has historically been viewed as the most 'risky' area in maternity care. Clements (2001) believes that there are two factors which make the labour suite a particularly vulnerable setting.

1. Public expectation – if a 'previously fit and healthy young woman' having a baby is 'injured' in the process she is much more likely to sue than is a patient being treated for a severe illness.
2. Monetary compensation for a 'brain damaged baby' can now reach £5 million (*CD* v. *Sefton Health Authority* [2004]) and attracts great media attention.

The challenge was to introduce a system where all members of the multidisciplinary team could participate in a non-threatening environment in analysis of incidents reported.

Guidelines for the 'Dos and Don'ts of Real Time' were formulated which addressed the issues of confidentiality and the importance of a non-judgmental approach in the examination of case notes, opinions on the decisions made and the outcomes for mother or baby. The mantra of Real Time became 'There is so much good in the worst of us and so much bad in the rest of us, that it doesn't do for any of us to sit and judge the rest of us' (Anon). Retrospective analysis as with the Perinatal Meetings when a poor outcome may already be known may lead to biased interpretation of the decision-making process in the case. Staff were reminded at the start of Real Time that the retrospectoscope always works better than any other scope. There was an opportunity at these daily meetings to explore and appreciate the many different roles and responsibilities of the individual practitioners who work together to provide a safe and satisfying maternity care service.

Meaningful feedback to staff from incident reporting has always been a problem; when incidents disappear into a management 'black hole', this does not encourage either participation in risk management nor learning from events (Cozens-Firth et al 2004, Knight 2004). Lessons learned from incident reporting in the early stages of incident reporting were compiled into a booklet called 'Midwifery and obstetric problems – did you know?' (SCRH 2004). This is updated on a yearly basis and has been distributed to all staff and is included in the new staff induction programme.

Another problem for staff is 'What to report?' (Cozens-Firth et al 2004). The use of trigger events or what to report lists are now available and these were used to highlight what events should be reported (RCOG 2005). Laminated copies of these lists were displayed in the labour suite. The incident reports (paper) were collated by the night staff along with the women's notes. Dependent on the activity on the labour suite and the volume of elective work (e.g. elective caesarean sections), 'Real Time' was called and all available staff met in the resource room (an area on the labour suite where posters, videos and simulation materials were available for staff's continuing clinical education). A record of attendees was kept and this demonstrated participation from obstetric consultants, midwives, clinical support workers (CSWs – who work under the auspices of the midwives when providing basic care), medical and midwifery students, senior obstetricians and junior obstetricians. Many staff were keen to use participation as evidence of their continued professional development and consulted the attendance records prior to appraisal.

Where appropriate, theatre staff from the adjoining theatre and anaesthetic staff attended. A feedback book was kept, recording the issues discussed and recommendations made, and risk summaries were produced by the Clinical Risk Coordinator. Thus staff who were not able to remain at the end of their shift could access the results of the discussions.

A questionnaire asking staff about their views on feedback undertaken in January 2004 revealed that the preferred method of feedback of incidents was either on a one-to-one basis with the Clinical Risk Coordinator or the weekly summaries or risk alerts produced by the Clinical Risk Coordinator (McNally 2005). Ideally the staff who reported the incident were encouraged to present their own incidents but with $12\frac{1}{2}$-hour shifts this was not always achievable.

It became apparent over time that an incident discussed at Real Time could be presented at other local meetings such as the Perinatal Meeting, the Perinatal Mortality Audit Meeting and the CTG Meetings.

At one Real Time an obstetrician presented her third incidence of third degree tear and asked those gathered on their experiences and strategies in reducing/preventing perineal trauma. Following meetings, the Clinical Risk Coordinator on a regular basis ensures that clinical support workers and students understand what is being discussed and is available to clarify any points that they do not understand. On the occasion mentioned, a CSW expressed her surprise that a 'doctor should ask for help and advice from colleagues' as she always thought 'doctors were gods'. She asked if this view could be communicated to the public at large so that they could appreciate that doctors are human and do make mistakes. They come to work to do a good job and reflect with others on how to continuously improve their practice.

The five top incidents discussed at Real Time to date have been:

1. unexpected admission of a term baby without major congenital abnormalities to the neonatal unit
2. major postpartum haemorrhage
3. arterial umbilical cord gas less than pH 7.1
4. shoulder dystocia
5. third/fourth degree perineal tear

Among the 700 staff in the SCRH there were many who had attended the Advanced Life Support in Obstetrics course (ALSO 1999). There are at least 12 members of staff who were designated ALSO instructors – a reflection of the teaching expertise within the unit. Among the obstetricians several have undertaken

Management of Obstetric Emergencies and Trauma (MOET).

At Real Time many of the mnemonics and acronyms from the ALSO course became integrated into the lessons learnt and risk summaries.

The Dr C Bravado mnemonic as recommended by CESDI (1999) was used to highlight the risks of ignoring the pattern of uterine activity and the dangers to mothers and fetus of hyper-stimulation with syntocinon in augmented and induced labours. When case notes were reviewed for a low cord pH or the unexpected admission of a baby to the neonatal unit with suspected hypoxic ischaemic encephalopathy there were often occasions where there was evidence of failure to assess the uterine contractions and resting tone in conjunction with the fetal heart rate. The use of the Dr C Bravado mnemonic is emphasised at all meetings where CTG interpretation is undertaken and this systematic approach prompts all staff to consider the contractions as part of every CTG assessment. The use of the mnemonic can be monitored as part of a documentation audit.

The mnemonic prompts staff to answer the following points when assessing a CTG trace:

DR	→ <u>D</u>efine <u>R</u>isk. High or low risk
C	is the woman <u>C</u>ontracting?
BRA	→ what is the <u>B</u>aseline <u>RA</u>te?
V	→ what is the <u>V</u>ariability (>5–10, <5–10)?
A	→ are there <u>A</u>ccelerations present?
D	→ are there <u>D</u>ecelerations present?
O	→ document <u>O</u>verall assessment as reassuring or non-reassuring trace and document action plan

The HELPERR mnemonic was also employed to ensure all staff were aware of the importance of a consistent, evidence-based, multidisciplinary approach to shoulder dystocia – and the importance of good record keeping and timeous documentation of manoeuvres employed:

H	→ call for <u>H</u>elp
E	→ evaluate need for an <u>E</u>pisiotomy
L	→ <u>L</u>egs into McRobert's manoeuvre
P	→ suprapubic <u>P</u>ressure

E → Enter hands into vagina to perform internal manoeuvres

R → Remove the posterior arm

R → Roll the mother onto all fours.

At Real Time community midwives were often present in the labour suite as part of rotation. They would often share their experiences of home births and would recommend that the all fours position should be used first as they found positional changes such as this were much more effective in preventing dystocia.

The use of Dr C Bravado and the HELPERR mnemonics were reviewed at Real Time. Examples of exemplary practice were also presented at the meetings. Risk management and incident reporting should include the positive aspects of care as well as the care delivery problems identified. Where care management problems were identified or sub-optimal care suspected these were referred to locally as PFI (potential for improvement). Individuals whose practice was thought to be in need of PFI were followed up by either the Clinical Risk Coordinator or through the Supervisors of Midwives system or through the educational supervisor system for medical staff.

Postpartum haemorrhage may be a feature in the labour suite. The SCRH adopted the advice of Professor Drife on what to do when this occurs: 'Use the Tarrant manoeuvre – phone a friend' (Drife 2001).

This advice stressed to staff that in a particularly busy teaching hospital all staff should feel empowered to seek advice/call for help early and where practice deficiencies were identified to ask for more supervised practice.

The trigger for reporting postpartum haemorrhage was blood loss in excess of 1000 ml. Recently the unit has been contributing to a Scottish audit of severe maternal morbidity and has adopted its criteria for major obstetric haemorrhage. The labour suite uses a combination of a 'pathophysiological' (or clinically based) and 'management based' definitions. (An example of a clinically based definition is estimated blood loss of more than 2500 ml; an example of a management based definition is transfused with more than five units of blood.) All incidents of haemorrhage were analysed, with particular emphasis on early recognition of the cause of the haemorrhage which could have major implications on the management of the haemorrhage.

Staff were urged to ask themselves if the haemorrhage was due to the 'Four Ts':

Tone: atonic haemorrhage
Trauma: traumatic haemorrhage
Tissue: retained placental tissue
Thrombin: coagulation disorders

This helped to minimise the use of syntocinon for perineal and cervical bleeding where the use of syntocinon was not indicated in the presence of a well contracted uterus. It also prompted staff to consider an evacuation of uterus sooner rather than later thus reducing the risk of continued blood loss.

Real Time incident reporting has now been a feature in the SCRH for 4 years. Other areas in maternity were keen to introduce this learning from incident reporting approach, and since 2005 there have been fortnightly meetings on the Neonatal Unit. The postnatal wards have a period of their staff meetings dedicated to incident reporting. If, however, an incident is considered serious or where immediate action and investigation are required (severe maternal/newborn morbidity or mortality) staff follow a flowchart for the escalation of serious incidents so that the Clinical Director (medical), the Principal Midwife and senior hospital management are aware of the event.

One of the trigger events that indicate when an incident form should be completed is either an unexpected return to theatre or unexpected return to the High Dependency Unit (HDU) on the labour suite. Secondary postpartum haemorrhage (within 12–24 hours of delivery) was identified as one of the most common causes. An analysis of care identified that there was an apparent lack of the appreciation of the unique haemorrhage response of fit healthy women to blood loss and/or hypovolaemic shock. 'Young, previously fit, pregnant women have significant physiological reserve in most organ systems. The effect of this is to mask the physiological signs of a number of important pathological conditions, most notably hypovolaemia and systemic sepsis' (CEMACH 2004: 237). Once more the service was able to audit its practice against the findings of the Confidential Enquiry (CEMACH 2004). It became apparent through incident analysis that staff did not realise that the population that they were caring for were able to compensate so well haemodynamically with blood loss that women were often moribund or very seriously ill before they were transferred to adult intensive care. An educational drive, comprising posters, presentations and teaching sessions was initiated to highlight that the pulse rather than the blood pressure (BP) is a better indicator of deterioration in fit, young women. The integrated care pathway (ICP) form for recovery and post-procedure observations was amended to highlight the importance of monitoring the pulse, a woman's pallor and her peripheries and the significance of palpating the abdomen for signs of swelling which could signify intraabdominal bleeding.

A helpful acronym was developed and is displayed in all clinical areas. It is referred to as the 'Seven Ps'.

P pulse
P peripheries
P pallor
P abdominal distension or pain
P blood pressure
P bleeding per vaginam
P puncture – bloods taken for heamacue and full blood count and coagulation studies

The hospital as a whole is implementing a scoring guide for the detection of 'at risk patients'. 'Hospitals should have a track and trigger system that allows rapid detection of the signs of early clinical deterioration and an early and appropriate response' (NCEPOD 2005). The scoring system will be adapted to suit the special needs of ill women in maternity. It is referred to in the literature as Systemic Early Warning System (SEWS).

One of the strengths of incident reporting is that it can highlight trends which may on analysis reveal an educational need and a need for awareness raising among staff.

Along with the changes to practice mentioned previously there was one other major change where the findings from incident analysis and case review have resulted in action which will in the future be published nationwide. This was an attempt to reduce the incidence of babies admitted to the neonatal unit with hypernatraemic dehydration of the newborn.

In 2001 the maternity unit won the prestigious UNICEF Baby Friendly award in recognition of its high standards in supporting breastfeeding. At the same time, incident reporting highlighted a number of babies readmitted with weight loss and high sodium levels. These babies were all almost exclusively breast-fed. In response to the admission rate the Clinical Risk Coordinator and Infant Feeding Strategist aimed to help parents and midwives recognise the signs of ineffective feeding, launch educational sessions on strategies to overcome ineffective feeding and devise a system where midwives could have direct referral for babies not responding to these strategies. A Jaundice and Weight Loss clinic was established on the Neonatal Unit and midwives could directly refer parents and babies to be seen if they found that their strategies to overcome ineffective feeding were not working.

Audit has shown that the number of babies being referred fluctuates from month to month, however, the overall serum sodium levels of babies referred to the clinic is reducing. In early 2000 levels were being recorded at 170–180 mmol/l. Over the past 2 years there have been very few serum sodium levels recorded over the upper limit of the normal of 140 mmol/l, which points to the success of early recognition of a problem and early intervention.

Early recognition on the postnatal wards of feeding problems is communicated to the community midwives so that as part of planning their daily workload they can identify women who will require extra help.

In the last 3 years, the SCRH has:

1. Designed the leaflet 'How to know your baby is getting enough milk'. This has proven very

popular with mothers and midwives and has been sought after by many other midwifery units. The National Childbirth Trust is working with the Infant Feeding Strategist and the Clinical Risk Coordinator to produce a leaflet which will be available throughout the UK in the near future.

2. Ensured every mother receives a copy of the leaflet.
3. Ensured that mothers are shown how to hand express and cup feed their babies when necessary (i.e. when baby is not feeding effectively).
4. And finally, guidelines have been developed for midwives on recognising and helping the reluctant feeder.

MEASURES INTRODUCED TO REDUCE RISK AND WHERE THIS SITS WITH WOMEN'S CHOICE IN PREGNANCY AND CHILDBIRTH

Many practices have been implemented in the SCRH in response to the ever increasing awareness of the need to reduce risks in maternity, as well as to improve outcomes and reduce litigation claims. However there are times when women's choices may conflict with recommended practices to reduce risk. Some examples from this inner city teaching hospital are explored here.

1. Cord pH
2. Perineal and abdominal suturing
3. External cephalic version (ECV)
4. Home birth with the potential for complications

CORD pH

Apgar scores of less than 5 at 5 minutes and a cord pH of less than 7.1 are reportable incidents in the SCRH. The presence of the findings of low Apgar scores at 5 minutes and a low cord pH may assist in excluding an intrapartum cause for any subsequent neurological deficit. Cord samples are taken for all babies at the SCRH. From a risk management perspective

this is considered good practice. Parents are not asked routinely for consent nor are they given any choice in the matter. When a low cord pH is recorded the 'Protocol for low cord pH' is followed. This entails paediatric review and a repeat blood gas hours later. However midwives are increasingly questioning the defensive nature of this routine, especially when the baby is in good condition at birth (Shallow 2003). More recently women have asked that cord gases are not performed as they do not wish to know the pH and do not want the planned intervention should a low cord pH be recorded. As choice implies access to information, the unit is considering giving women the information concerning the risks and the questions surrounding the benefits of cord pH measurements.

PERINEAL AND ABDOMINAL SUTURING

Many mothers with access to the internet are questioning the suturing of second degree tears following a spontaneous vertex delivery. Many wish that secondary healing should take place and choose not to have their perineum sutured. Many of the midwives have attended study days on perineal trauma and its management. The recommendation now is that almost all second degree tears should be sutured to reduce risks at a later date of poor alignment at the fourchette and possible dyspareunia.

Practice may be becoming driven by protocols and guidelines. This may be due to the influence of validating bodies such as the CNST which, when they visit hospitals, look for evidence of policies, procedures and guidelines for many aspects of practice which formerly were reserved to the judgment of the individual professional. The presence of policies, etc. may mean that hospitals, by demonstrating compliance with CNST requirements, may receive a reduction in their negligence indemnity insurance premium. Many professionals may feel that this encourages a more litigation-minded approach to reducing risk and ignores the role of women's informed choice on many clinical matters.

On the other hand, there has been much debate on the use of single layer suturing as opposed to multiple closure of each layer in the closure of the abdomen following caesarean section. Some women's support groups are encouraging women to exercise choice and state which form of closure they would prefer. Can woman really exercise this degree of choice in matters of major surgery?

EXTERNAL CEPHALIC VERSION

In order to reduce the trend towards elective caesarean section for all breech presentations, maternity units in the UK have been urged to have ECV clinics where the fetus is turned from breech to cephalic, making a vaginal delivery more possible. At the SCRH there is a weekly ECV clinic on the Labour Suite. Over the past 3 years many women have chosen not to accept the offer of an ECV, and instead elect to have a caesarean section. There are many internet sources describing the increased relative safety of elective caesarean section and the 'dangers' of a vaginal breech birth. There is evidence that women who have repeat caesarean sections may be predisposed to developing placenta praevia and placenta accreta in subsequent pregnancies. An exploration of this likelihood is often explained to women but overwhelmingly they appear to accept these risks. Once more how far can women exercise this degree of choice? There may be a feeling of 'it will not happen to me' and the risk of severe morbidity or even death may be seen as 'shroud waving' by the professionals.

HOME BIRTH WITH THE POTENTIAL FOR COMPLICATIONS

Many women choose home birth rather than giving birth in a large maternity hospital. In low risk women this is a safe and very satisfying option for them and their families. But many professionals, both medical and midwifery, consider that the potential for swift onset life-threatening events to occur for mother and fetus make this a very 'risky' choice. In the community setting around the SCRH the home birth rate has in certain areas increased.

Recently, women with risk factors (e.g. previous shoulder dystocia, previous postpartum haemorrhage or a haemoglobin level below 10 mg/dl) which health professionals may consider should preclude women from having a home birth, are choosing to accept the risks. Women's perception of acceptable risk and the differing one of the professionals is frequently a great 'bone of contention'. There may still exist a prevailing attitude among the professionals that women's acceptance of risk is not valid, despite women clearly taking responsibility for their chosen actions.

FUTURE CHALLENGES FOR RISK MANAGEMENT AND INCIDENT REPORTING IN THE MATERNITY SERVICES

In 2004 the SCRH adopted a paperless, electronic incident reporting system. This has necessitated ongoing teaching sessions on its use and fears over confidentiality are still expressed by many staff. There has been a reduction on the number of incidents reported but as there were, using the paper form, a lot of incidents submitted which were communication problems best dealt with by clinicians themselves at a local level, this has begun to even out.

Staff are encouraged to report incidents where shared learning among the multidisciplinary team could improve practice. Staff have been issued with a paper on 'Incidents which must be reported' so that serious incidents can be captured and analysed as soon as possible after the event. Major incidents are now subject to the process of Root Cause Analysis where all aspects of the event are explored (Taylor-Adams & Vincent 2004) This includes an individual's knowledge and experience, contributory factors such as team dynamics, work/environment and level of activity in the practice area at the time of the incident. Organisational systems are analysed and action planning is undertaken to ensure that learning has taken place and to reduce the risk of recurrence.

In some incidents a complaint or claim may be likely or almost certain to occur. The

Clinical Risk Coordinator is charged with obtaining statements from the staff involved so that when memories have faded after the event or staff have moved away there is a record of the events readily available. Writing statements and indeed participating in Root Cause Analysis is often a very stressful and worrying time for staff. A future challenge for risk management and incident reporting is to make this process an acceptable part of the culture of accountability and not a finger pointing, 'scapegoating' or blaming exercise as it is often perceived.

As the primary role of the Supervisor of Midwives is to protect the public from the consequences of poor practice, in the future they will be more involved in ensuring learning from incidents has taken place and participate in supporting midwives through the Root Cause Investigatory process.

CONCLUSION

Some staff have referred to Risk Management and Incident Reporting as the 'new kid on the block' suggesting that it is a 'fad', a fashion that will soon be replaced by yet another. However the climate where patient safety is paramount on everyone's agenda is showing no signs of abating. There is, however, a concurrent rise in consumer participation in discussion of choices available, and in an increasing litigious environment in maternity care, risk reducing strategies implemented by the professionals may be seen as an attempt to stifle that right to choose and as leading to more defensive practice.

George Bernard Shaw said 'All professions are a conspiracy against the laity' and this is indeed how some of the consumers inputting in the management of the maternity services at the SCRH view risk reducing measures on occasions. Further discussion of the role of risk management and opportunities it affords inpatient safety and choice may reduce this cynicism.

The experiences in the SCRH of risk management and incident reporting has meant that in the future they will be seen to be less the preserve of an individual or a department but activities embedded in everyone's day-to-day practice. Staff will be more and more accountable for continuously improving the care they provide supported by the concept of institutional Clinical Governance.

Legal Case

CD v. Sefton Health Authority [2004]. Online. Available: http://www.jmw-clinical-negligence.co.uk/athetoid_cerebral_palsy.html

References

ALSO (Advanced Life Support in Obstetrics) 1999 Course Syllabus. American Academy of Family Physicians, Leawood, Kansas

CEMACH (Confidential Enquires into Maternal and Child Health) 2004 Why mothers die 2000–2002. RCOG Press, London. Online. Available: www.cemach.org.uk

CEMD 1999 Why mothers die 1997–1999. Maternal and Child Health Consortium, London

CESDI (Confidential Enquiry into Stillbirth and Deaths in Infancy) 1999 Confidential enquiry into stillbirth and deaths in infancy. Maternal and Child Health Consortium, London

Chambers R, Wakley G 2000 Making clinical governance work for you. Radcliffe Medical Press, Oxford

Clements RV (ed) 2001 Risk management and litigation in obstetrics and gynaecology. Royal Society of Medicine Press, London

Cooper IG 2000 Clinical risk management in professional studies for midwifery practice. Churchill Livingstone, Edinburgh

Cozens-Firth J, Redfern N, Moss F 2004 Confronting errors in patient care: the experiences of doctors and nurses. Clinical Risk 10(5): 184–190

Currie L, Morrell C, Scrivener R 2004 Clinical governance: quality at the centre of services. British Journal of Midwifery 12(5): 330–334

DH 2000 An organisation with a memory: a report of an expert advisory group on learning from adverse events in the NHS. The Stationery Office, London

Drife J 2001 Reducing the risk in obstetrics. In: Vincent C (ed) Clinical risk management, 2nd edn. BMJ Publishing Group, London

Green S 2001 Benefiting from the end of the blame culture. Professional Nurse 16(7): S3–S4

Kingston MJ, Evans SM, Smith BJ et al 2004 Attitudes of doctors and nurses towards incident reporting: a qualitative analysis. Medical Journal of Australia 181(1): 36–39

Knight D 2004 Incident reporting: every nurse's responsibility. Paediatric Nursing 16: 23–27

Lilley 1999 Making sense of clinical governance: a workbook for NHS doctors, nurses and managers. Radcliffe Medical Press, Oxford

McNally S 2005 Staff perception of incident reporting and risk management. (Unpublished Staff Survey, Lothian NHS)

NCEPOD (National Confidential Enquiry into Patient Outcome and Death) 2005 Recommendations. In: NCEPOD report 2005. Online. Available: http://www.ncepod.org.uk/2005report/recommendations.html

NPSA (National Patient Safety Agency) 2004 Seven steps to patient safety: an overview guide for NHS staff. National Patient Safety Agency, London. Online. Available: http://www.npsa.nhs.uk/site/media/documents/499_sevensteps_overview(2).pdf

Quinn M 2003 Reality management: real time data let hospital leaders base decisions on what's happening now, not last year. Trustee 56(5): 8–12, 1

Reason JT 2001 Understanding adverse events: the human factor. In: Vincent C (ed) Clinical risk management, 2nd edn. British Institute Medical Journal Books, London

RCOG (Royal College of Obstetricians and Gynaecologists) 2005 Improving patient safety: risk management for maternity and gynaecology. Clinical Governance Advice No 2, October. RCOG, London

Richardson C 2002 Slow progress on the no-blame culture. Health Care Risk Report, 8(5): 20–21

SCRH (Simpson Centre for Reproductive Health) 2004 Midwifery/obstetric problems: did you know . . .? NHS Lothian, Edinburgh

Shallow H 2003 Should cord pH be performed routinely after normal birth? RCM Midwives 6(1): 28–31

Simpson KR 2000 Creating a culture of safety: a shared responsibility. Maternal and Child Nursing 25(2): 61

SPCERH (Scottish Programme for Clinical Effectiveness in Reproductive Health) 2004 Annual report

Taylor-Adams S, Vincent C (2004) Systems analysis of clinical incidents: the London Protocol. Clinical Risk 10(6): 211–220

Chapter 7

Risk and Choice: Remote and Rural Risk Issues in the UK

Lesley Anne Smith

INTRODUCTION

GENERAL

Risk management is a component part of Clinical Governance which aims to ensure patients receive safe and up-to-date clinical care. It is important to manage the risks which exist within a healthcare setting in order to:

- reduce and, as far as possible, eliminate harm to patients
- improve the quality of care
- minimise the impact of adverse events on the staff, finances, reputation and objectives of the organisation
- ensure that lessons are learnt and that the resulting solutions are shared as widely as possible

The term 'clinical risk management' is sometimes used to refer to the application of risk management in the clinical setting. However the distinction between 'clinical' and 'non-clinical' risk is often blurred and analysis of an adverse event may show that both types of risk have been involved. This chapter will discuss the application of maternity care risk management within the context of a remote and rural setting. It will note how choices are made, and how consultation and dialogue are key elements in providing effective care.

ELEMENTS OF RISK MANAGEMENT

The basic steps of risk management, which can be applied at any level of an organisation, are as follows:

- **Consultation** or communication with a wide variety of stakeholders
- **Establish the context** in which the rest of the process will take place
- **Identification** or recognition of major risks
- **Analysis of the risks** to determine the likelihood and consequence and hence the level of risk
- **Evaluation** of these risks to establish how serious they are and determine a priority for dealing with them
- **Control** of the risks by preparing an Action Plan
- **Monitoring** and review of the process

Risk management should be a proactive process which assesses potential risks and reduces them to a level as low as is reasonably practicable. It plays a vital role in supporting and informing decision-making in providing a safe and secure environment for patients, staff and visitors (AS/NZS 2004).

RISK MANAGEMENT WITHIN MATERNITY CARE

Maternity care is a recognised high-risk clinical specialty primarily because if things do go wrong the severity of the outcome can be very significant – death of mother or baby or significant brain injury to the child.

These factors have been recognised by obstetricians, gynaecologists and midwives and there are several publications from professional bodies making recommendations in relation to clinical governance issues, risk management practices, revalidation, etc. For example:

- Royal College of Obstetricians and Gynaecologists, Royal College of Midwives. Towards Safer Childbirth – Minimum Standards for the Organisation of the Labour Ward (RCOG/RCM 1999): makes a number of recommendations regarding staffing of labour wards, communications and education and training standards.
- Royal College of Obstetricians and Gynaecologists. Clinical Governance Advice No 2.: Clinical Risk Management for Obstetricians and Gynaecologists (RCOG 2001): a practical approach to clinical risk management which might be adopted at the level of an individual maternity unit, or a group of departments within a Health Board region.

A national expert working group on acute maternity services (EGAMS) was set up by the Scottish Executive and reported in December 2002. The report of this expert group stated:

The present provision and shape of acute maternity services is no longer sustainable in the light of changes in the number and locations of births in Scotland (demographic changes), training, and workforce pressures and the need to ensure clinically safe and cost-effective care.

(SEHD 2002a)

The EGAMS report describes eight levels of maternity care, and specifies the risk management and staff competencies required at each level, to ensure the safest possible outcome for mother and baby. The issues addressed in the report are particularly relevant in remote and rural areas and maternity services in many areas of Scotland are being reviewed as a result.

The Scottish Executive recently published the Kerr Report which considers the future shape of the National Health Service (NHS) in Scotland (SEHD 2005). The recommendations set out in this report were guided by a number of factors including rural issues and patient expectation and public trust. The report recognises that rural communities face particular challenges in terms of transport, access to services and the sustainability of local communities and that any model of care must meet these rural needs. Alongside this is the public and patients' expectation that services can be accessed as quickly as possible, be of consistently high standards and delivered by suitably trained professionals.

EXAMPLE OF MATERNITY CARE IN A REMOTE AND RURAL SETTING

The Highlands of Scotland comprise the largest and most sparsely populated part of the UK with all the attendant issues of a difficult terrain and a limited internal transport and communications infrastructure. The area covers almost 25 784 km² (10 000 square miles), which represents approximately one third of the Scottish land surface.

NHS Highland serves a population of some 208 000 residents and a proportion of its patients result from the influx of tourists to the Highlands, which at certain times of the year can double or even triple the local population. The city of Inverness is the largest urban area in the region with a population of around 60 000. The majority of the population, however, lives in rural areas which may be remote, including islands. The geographical nature of the region presents particular challenges for the efficient and effective delivery of healthcare services.

There is a district general hospital (DGH) in Inverness which has over 550 beds and which provides specialist care for the highland population. This includes a consultant-led specialist maternity unit where about 1800 babies are born each year, and which has an on-site 11-cot neonatal facility. In addition there is a consultant-led obstetric unit in Wick, which is over 100 miles north of Inverness, and there are community maternity units based in Fort William, approximately 80 miles to the southwest, and on the Isle of Skye, off the west coast of the mainland (Fig. 7.1). A network of community midwives supports the delivery of maternity care throughout the region.

The remoteness and rurality of the area results in specific challenges for the staff who are providing care in these areas. These include the differing roles within the wider rural maternity team, staff competence and confidence in clinical practice and issues around skills maintenance and training. These factors need to be taken into account in supporting and informing

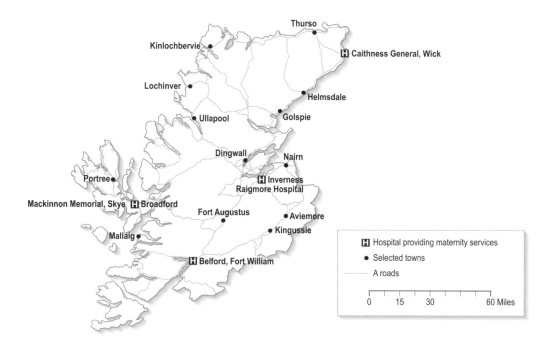

Figure 7.1

Case Study

The following fictional case study brings together some of the themes which will be explored in the remainder of this chapter.

Mrs A is a 30-year-old para 1+0 who lives on a small island off the coast of Scotland. Her son was born 18 months previously, following an uncomplicated pregnancy. He was delivered at term in a large maternity unit on the mainland and Mrs A was relatively happy with the care she received.

The island is 20 miles from the mainland and is served by a ferry which runs three times a week. Local health services consist of a surgery held twice a week by a general practitioner (GP) and a triple duty nurse (combined District Nurse, Midwife and Health Visitor) who travel from the mainland. No health professionals live on the island.

Mrs A's husband is a fisherman who often spends several days at a time away at sea.

When Mrs A attended her first antenatal appointment in the peripatetic GP surgery she informed the midwife that she had decided to have a home birth.

What are the factors which now need to be considered?

The first thing to say is that Mrs A has exercised her right to choose the place of birth. The position of choice within the provision of the maternity services has been integral since the seminal Changing Childbirth report in England and Wales (DH 1993) and its Scottish equivalent, the Scottish Policy Review (Scottish Office 1993). The more recent Framework for Maternity Services in Scotland report (Scottish Executive 2001: 13) states that 'Women have the right to choose how and where they give birth.' The Kerr Report also recognises the importance of choice, stating that 'a service which is built around choice is likely to meet more what users want, and to have higher levels of satisfaction.' Such rights have to be achieved in real life settings, of course, and there are particular factors when trying to do this in a remote or rural setting. One of these is to evaluate the relevant risk factors.

decision-making in providing a safe and secure environment for patients, staff and visitors.

RISK ASSESSMENT IN A REMOTE AND RURAL SETTING

CONSULTATION AND COMMUNICATION

One of the first steps in carrying out a risk assessment of any service or individual case is identification of the risks involved. Some of the risk factors will be easily identifiable but others may be less obvious. It is therefore important that as wide a range of staff are involved in this process as possible to ensure that all possible risks are identified. Equally important is the involvement of service users in this process. This can occur either at the individual level, where a woman is involved in the discussions of the risk factors in relation to her specific situation, or at a community level where the public is involved in decisions about service change.

It must always be remembered that patients have a fundamental legal and ethical right to determine what happens to their own body. Valid consent to treatment is therefore absolutely central in all forms of healthcare, from providing personal care to undertaking major surgery. Seeking consent is also a matter of common courtesy between health professionals and patients. A patient must be properly informed about the risks, benefits and consequences of any proposed treatment and possible alternatives before signing a consent form. A fully informed patient is less likely to have cause to complain or to resort to litigation (DH 2001).

The Department of Health (DH) published a strategy in 2004 which recognises that better healthcare outcomes are achieved when the partnership between patient and health professional is at its strongest (DH 2004). The strategy aims to improve access for all to the quality general and personalised information people need and want in order to exercise choice about their personal health and healthcare.

The Scottish Executive Health Department (SEHD) issued guidance in 2004 on how staff within SEHD and NHS Scotland should involve, engage and consult the public from the outset when any service changes are being proposed (SEHD 2004a). This guidance states that effective public involvement should promote wider acceptance by people and communities of the need for service change and increase public confidence and trust. It stresses that end-stage consultation is not enough.

RISK IDENTIFICATION

In general, risk factors can be grouped into three main categories:

- Human factors
- Equipment related factors
- Organisational factors

Some examples are considered below specifically in relation to remote and rural issues.

Human Factors

Clinical Cover in an Emergency

When any model of care provision is being assessed it is necessary to consider what would happen in an emergency situation should specialist staff not be available. In relation to midwifery care, those women with identifiable clinical risk factors should be considered for delivery in a specialist unit. However, it must always be acknowledged that pregnancy, particularly delivery, can be unpredictable and unforeseen emergencies require to be coped with. In the case study referred to above, for instance, it would be appropriate to establish which practitioners might be required in order to cope with an emergency, and how they would be organised in order to do so effectively.

This in itself brings additional factors into consideration, which are discussed further in the following paragraphs.

Experience and Competence

A number of issues have emerged over the past few years which have called into question the viability of specialist-led obstetric services in more remote and rural areas. These include national medical workforce issues including the move towards increasing sub-specialisation (SEHD 2002b); the impact of complying with the European Working Times Directive, which limits the time that staff are available for on-call commitments (The Working Time Regulations 1999 (S.I. No. 3372), and the Working Time (Amendment) Regulations 2001 (S.I. No. 3256) are examples of legislation originating from the European Union, which have set limits on the number of hours people can work); the difficulties associated with skill maintenance in units with low and falling birth rates; and implementation of new contractual arrangements for medical staff which are designed to formalise working hours and to enable efficient and effective use of consultant time (DH 2003, SEHD 2004b).

Similar concerns relate to other groups of staff including midwives, paramedics, anaesthetists and general surgeons. Changes to working practices and the impact of clinical standards may result in units seeing only a limited number of complex cases. Maintaining skills and competence in specialist areas can be difficult in these circumstances.

Training

Many of the above issues are linked to the availability and accessibility of training. Working in a remote area can mean that it is difficult to access appropriate training courses. A lack of local courses means that staff are required to travel to attend courses with the result that training can become costly both in financial terms and in terms of staff time. This has an obvious personal effect but can also have a wider impact on the care which can be provided if staff are required to be away from their place of work for a considerable period of time with limited cover available.

Communication

It is well recognised that lack of communication can contribute significantly to adverse events (NPSA 2005). Situations which require the transfer of a pregnant woman/newly delivered mother and baby between units or from the community to the hospital setting require careful consideration. Particular communication issues may arise in the emergency situation where there are no specialist staff on site.

Staffing Levels and Shift Patterns

The impact of remoteness is particularly felt in relation to staffing levels and the requirements to be on call. Community midwives who are on call for a home confinement, for example, may find that they are required to be available for a considerable period of time with no break, thus contravening Working Time regulations. In addition, transfers of emergency cases to the larger centre may require the one specialist who is available for the area to accompany the woman, thus leaving the area with no cover. These considerations require to be taken into account when planning staffing levels, designing rotas and developing contingency plans to cover emergency situations.

Equipment Related Factors

Much of the care which is provided by health professionals is dependent on having the correct equipment. Risks arise when equipment is either not available or is inappropriate for the job in hand, when equipment fails or when staff have not been adequately trained in its use.

The issues relating to training have been explored above. Staff familiarity with equipment is very important and this can be compromised if different models of the same equipment are in use in different units in the region. This may result from an uncoordinated approach to equipment purchase, the resolution of which may take several years due to the costs of the equipment involved.

Consideration must always be given to the requirements to adequately maintain equipment thus reducing the chances of it failing during use. This is especially important in small units and community settings where there may only be one of that particular item available. For some pieces of equipment local staff can be trained to carry out these regular checks, but more complex medical equipment may need to be maintained or repaired by specialist staff. Some of these items, such as Entonox or Oxygen Regulators and Fetal Dopplers, can be sent to the specialist centre, whereas other items such as incubators and cardiotocography (CTG) machines may well require the specialist to travel to the local setting.

Organisational Factors

Environment

Transport issues are a major concern for both staff and patients and their relatives. Many remote communities are a considerable distance from the main hospital sites, often along single-track roads. These risks can be compounded by bad weather, especially in the winter months. Public transport services also have to be considered in relation to the availability of bus and rail services. Availability of ambulance transport is another major concern, especially in smaller communities: transport of an emergency to the major hospital may leave the community without further ambulance cover.

The impact of patients being looked after in hospitals distant from their home always requires to be considered. In relation to midwifery care, planned admission to a specialist unit for delivery may require the woman to be away from home for several days in advance of the birth. Accommodation will therefore have to be provided close to the hospital. In addition, the woman's partner and other children may also require accommodation around the time of the birth and in the case of emergency transfers, this may be needed at short notice.

Interaction of Teams

In many areas there is a move to an integrated model of midwifery service. This means bringing together the community and hospital midwifery staff into one team with a single leadership structure and common service standards. Many remote and rural areas are served by a double or triple duty nurse, and integrating these complex roles can provide a particular challenge.

It is clear from the above that there may be times when the health professionals' assessment of the risks associated with any particular case conflict with the choices which the individual patient wishes to make. It is therefore important to consider the next stage of the process, namely

Case Study (continued)

Mrs A's midwife noted her wish for a home birth but was unhappy about agreeing to this without first discussing it with the GP and with other colleagues including her Supervisor of Midwives.

During these discussions it was agreed that Mrs A's age, general health and previous maternal history meant that she fell into a 'low risk' category. However, staff were particularly concerned about three factors. The agreed standard was that for planned home births there should be two trained professionals present, one of whom is a midwife. In addition, as the ferry does not run every day, there was a risk that Mrs A could go into labour and trained staff would not be able to attend immediately. One way of addressing this risk would be for the identified staff to be permanently located on the island for a period of time prior to Mrs A's due date. The knock-on effect of both these factors would be to deplete the pool of staff available to staff the on-call rota on the mainland. The staff were also concerned that, although Mrs A was considered low risk, an unforeseen emergency could arise, putting the life of mother and baby at risk. It was agreed that the midwife should discuss these issues with Mrs A to see if she would agree to have her baby in the Midwifery Unit on the mainland.

an assessment of the risks in order to determine what is acceptable to the staff and to the patient or community and what is not.

EVALUATION OF THE IDENTIFIED RISKS

Once the risks have been identified the next step is to consider the likelihood (frequency) of the risk actually happening and then relate this to the potential impact (consequence) that this event would have on the organisation, patients and/or staff.

Likelihood

An assessment of the possible frequency of any event is based on the likelihood of loss, damage or injury arising from the risk identified. This can vary from an event being considered very rare, through to it being considered almost certain to occur.

Consequence

Once the likelihood or frequency is determined then the impact of the risk must be determined. This will reflect the impact on the individual or the organisation should an identified risk or event occur.

In relation to an individual woman or child the consequence of any risk may range from minimal harm through an increased length of stay in hospital, to permanent injury or even death.

In relation to a clinical service, the effect on the ability to provide the service, the reputation of the department and the ability to meet nationally agreed quality standards are some of the issues that need to be considered.

Risk Rating

Once the likelihood and severity of any event have been assessed it is possible to use a risk matrix to determine whether a risk is categorised as High, Medium or Low. This is very useful for communicating the level of risk and aiding understanding of the process. An example of such a matrix is shown in Table 7.1 (AS/NZS 2004).

Table 7.1   Risk rating matrix

Likelihood	Consequences/impact				
	Insignificant	Minor	Moderate	Major	Extreme
Almost certain	MEDIUM	HIGH	HIGH	VERY HIGH	VERY HIGH
Likely	MEDIUM	MEDIUM	HIGH	HIGH	VERY HIGH
Possible	LOW	MEDIUM	HIGH	HIGH	HIGH
Unlikely	LOW	LOW	MEDIUM	MEDIUM	HIGH
Rare	LOW	LOW	MEDIUM	MEDIUM	HIGH

It is also possible to rank risks according to their 'level' and this is a very useful way of producing a prioritised list of risks. Actions can then be considered and choices made in relation to the priority of the risks related to the resources required for their management.

Sometimes evidence or statistics are available regarding the frequency and severity of certain events and these should be taken into account when making the assessment. In other cases, however, there will be no specific quantitative evidence on which to make this assessment and the decisions will be subjective and based on the opinions and experience of the personnel involved in the assessment. While in theory the decision-making process is always a collaborative one, with clinical practitioners and the pregnant woman discussing options and possible courses of action, in practice the pregnant woman's scope for exercising her autonomy in this way is often limited. However, in situations where there is a lack of professional consensus about preferred management, she may in fact have a greater opportunity to exercise her right to choice.

MANAGING THE RISKS

The next stage in the process is to consider what actions are required to manage the risks which have been identified. It may be that the activity should be eliminated entirely because it is too dangerous, or else steps are required to reduce the risk to a more acceptable level. This might be done by introducing new policies and procedures, purchasing new equipment, providing specific training, improving work instructions or considering changes to environmental factors. In some cases, especially when a whole service has been assessed, it may be that investment is required in terms of staffing, building works or major pieces of equipment.

Case Study (continued)

At her next antenatal clinical appointment Mrs A and the midwife had a long discussion about the risks associated with her decision to have a home birth. The midwife explained that one of the major concerns related to the frequency of the ferry. It was possible that the appropriate staff would not be able to cross to the island when Mrs A went into labour which could have a major impact on the safety of both her and her baby. It was the midwife's view that this represented a high risk which could be compounded by Mr A being away at sea at the same time.

Mrs A accepted the midwife's view but she was concerned about who would look after her toddler son if she had to leave the island. She had no family living close by and did not wish him to be looked after by a neighbour. She remained adamant that she wished to have a home birth.

The midwife agreed to talk with the ferry company to see if it was possible for them to provide a ferry at short notice.

In this case it is possible to use the risk ranking process described above to assess any bids against others submitted to a planning and prioritisation process.

Examples of some of these in relation to the risks discussed earlier in the chapter are detailed below.

Policies and Procedures

To deal with emergency situations it is vital that unambiguous risk assessment protocols are in place. These protocols and supporting criteria will help the clinicians identify those patients who will require more intensive support than would be available locally. The written documents should be developed by the multidisciplinary team and should include specific information on who is responsible for carrying out key parts of the care or treatment, where that should be delivered and provide clear information on levels of accountability. Ideally these decisions should be made in a planned way so that women are cared for in the most appropriate setting for their needs. However, there will always be times when unexpected emergencies arise. In such circumstances having agreed protocols in place will ensure that consultant surgeons, anaesthetists and other professionals, as in all medical emergencies, are able to step in to ensure immediate stabilisation of the patient, be this the woman or the baby. An important component of these protocols is clear communication channels which ensure that clinical discussion can take place between the appropriate centres to determine the most appropriate action, e.g. immediate transfer, or transfer once the patient's condition is stable. It is also important to include the woman and/or her partner in any of these discussions. The EGAMS report (SEHD 2002a) recommends that clinical protocols for emergency interventions are regularly tested via risk assessment.

Training

When there are concerns about the ability of staff to maintain their level of skills, consideration can be given to development of clinical skills centres to offer continuing access to training modules, practice simulations, and IT links to an evidence database. These will ensure that staff are trained to cope with a wider range of more serious clinical interventions and have greater competencies in coping with obstetric and neonatal emergencies.

Where there are problems regarding the local availability of training courses, steps can be taken to address these issues by enhancing the role of midwifery educators to provide multidisciplinary training based on the needs of a particular locality. Developing rotational training programmes between different units within a region is another way of ensuring that staff are exposed to as wide a range of clinical situations as possible, especially if there is limited opportunity to experience such situations in their local unit. Support from other professionals such as neonatal nurse practitioners is also essential to ensure that midwives are comfortable with their competency, and that their practice is continuously updated.

As information technology continues to develop and become more widely available, staff should be encouraged to make use of online learning opportunities.

Staffing

Improvements to the care that can be provided to patients may result from the integration of midwifery teams across community and hospital settings. Given that any new model is likely to demand different levels of practice by the midwives, a Midwife Consultant post or an Area Senior Midwife post should be considered which would offer support in respect of clinical/professional leadership, research, audit and education, and would focus clinical practice at an advanced level.

Working Practices

Where there are concerns about staff working on their own a Lone Workers Policy should be considered. This can be supplemented by local systems which are established to ensure that somebody is aware of a staff member's whereabouts at all times. Mobile telephones have improved communications significantly but cannot always be relied upon in areas where coverage is poor.

Steps should be taken to ensure access to specialist staff, especially those who are off-site, via telephone and telemedicine links as appropriate.

Equipment

The provision of adequate levels of equipment which has been well maintained is vital in controlling any risks which patients and staff may be exposed to. Training in how to use any piece of equipment is also essential and this will be made much easier if the equipment in use throughout the area is of the same type – e.g. the same model of CTG machine.

The provision of a maintenance service for equipment being used in remote areas may best be achieved by way of a visiting service – a fully equipped van, visiting areas on a scheduled basis will reduce the need for equipment to be sent away and therefore reduces the

Case Study (continued)

The midwife contacted the ferry company and discussed the situation. The company confirmed that it would be possible to provide a ferry at short notice but that it would be for foot passengers only and not capable of carrying a car.

Following further discussion between the midwife, the GP and Mrs A, it was agreed to proceed with Mrs A's request for a home birth. Because the staff would not be able to take a car across to the island in an emergency, additional equipment which may be required was gathered together and stored at Mrs A's house. Changes were made to the on-call rota so that additional staff were available around the expected date of delivery. The GP and the midwife informed staff at the local rural community hospital of the situation and also contacted the specialist maternity unit. Mrs A made arrangements with her neighbour for the care of her son should this be necessary.

At 39 weeks Mrs A went into spontaneous labour and the two midwives who were on call travelled to the island without problem. Labour progressed, however the second stage was slower than anticipated. Mrs A delivered a large baby girl in good condition. Syntometrine 1 ml was administered by the first midwife as per the guidelines and the placenta and membranes were delivered within 5 minutes. The midwife checked the uterus was well contracted and the lochia appeared normal. Meanwhile, the second midwife had turned her attention to the baby and was preparing to help with breastfeeding when Mrs A complained of further bleeding.

The midwives recognised that Mrs A was having a significant postpartum haemorrhage (PPH) and the first midwife attempted to rub up a contraction and administered a further dose of syntometrine 1 ml in order to control the bleeding. The second midwife discussed the case with the GP, the rural community hospital and the maternity unit, and since the measures already taken were having little effect and the cause was established, the decision was taken to call the air ambulance and transfer to the specialist unit.

The midwives continued with interim measures as per guidelines. They also reassured Mrs A and her husband and helped with breastfeeding as this could also help to contract the uterus.

Following the decision to transfer, the midwives kept in regular contact with the consultant and the senior labour suite midwife in the maternity unit. The bleeding throughout was moderate and the midwives continued with the management of the situation. The helicopter arrived within an hour and Mrs A, the baby and the midwives were transferred directly to the maternity unit where Mrs A was assessed quickly and taken to theatre for an evacuation of retained products of conception (ERPC).

Mrs A and her daughter were discharged home 5 days later.

chances of it not being available when required.

It is important therefore to consider having in place an Equipment Replacement Strategy which is coordinated to ensure that the same type of equipment is purchased throughout the area. Staff should also be aware of how to report a faulty piece of equipment and how to get a replacement item if this is necessary. Special consideration should be given to contingency plans if there is only one of a particular item of equipment available in an area.

Environment

As discussed previously, one of the consequences of living in a remote area is that patients and their relatives may require to be treated in a unit distant from their home. This may require the provision of accommodation. It is important therefore to carry out an assessment of the availability and appropriateness of patient and family support accommodation to ensure it meets the needs of users and that it is of a modern standard and is family friendly.

MONITORING AND REVIEW

The final stage of the risk management process is to monitor and review the situation in order to assess whether the changes which have been introduced have had the desired effect on the identified risks.

CLINICAL INCIDENT RECORDING

One of the aims of clinical risk management is to reduce the frequency of adverse events and harm to patients (Clements 1995).

The presence of an adverse incident recording system is therefore one way in which the adequacy of any changes can be assessed. The type of incidents which are to be reported should be agreed by all the staff involved in the process and should be based on those incidents which pose the greatest risk to the mother or baby and from which the most lessons can be learnt.

An example of the types of incidents which may be reported is shown below:

- Unexpected poor condition of baby at birth; Apgar score less that 5 at 5 minutes; unexpected admission to Special Care Baby Unit
- Unexpected stillbirth
- Significant anomaly of baby noticed at birth
- Accidental trauma to mother or baby
- Maternal pathology, e.g. abruption, eclampsia, severe pre-eclamptic toxaemia
- PPH greater than 1500 ml
- Undiagnosed breech or twins
- Other (e.g. equipment failure, staff issues which affect patient care, re-admission with wound infection)

Should any of these incidents be reported, it is important that a brief outline of the clinical details of the case are also recorded. This will allow review of the case by a multidisciplinary group to assess what lessons can be learnt and what, if any, changes in practice are required to ensure that such incidents are less likely to occur in the future. There is also considerable benefit from discussing a selection of these cases with the wider maternity care team, and many departments hold regular Perinatal Morbidity and Mortality meetings for this purpose. Learning from adverse incidents is an important part of the process of continuous quality improvement. Clinical Governance arrangements should therefore be in place which include procedures for ensuring that information gained from adverse events is shared with the rest of the organisation as well as nationally, if appropriate, to improve service quality.

CLINICAL STANDARDS

Another method of monitoring improvements in clinical practice is to carry out repeat assessments of the service against published quality standards.

NHS Quality Improvement Scotland (NHS QIS) was set up by the Scottish Parliament in 2003 to take the lead in improving the quality of care and treatment delivered by NHS Scotland

Case Study (continued)

Mrs A's case was discussed at the multidisciplinary Perinatal Morbidity and Mortality meeting the following month. This was held at the specialist maternity unit and was attended by the community midwives and the GP.

It was agreed that the case had been well handled and that the outcome had therefore been positive as a result of the following:

- The midwives were competent and confident in managing this procedure because they had had regular skills training
- There were clear clinical guidelines on the management of PPH in the local area with which the midwife, GP, community hospital and the maternity unit were familiar
- Good communication was maintained between all those involved in the case, including Mrs A and her husband

(NHS QIS 2003). A major part of the remit of NHS QIS is to develop and run a national system of quality assurance of clinical services. Working in partnership with healthcare professionals and members of the public, NHS QIS sets standards for clinical services, assesses performance throughout NHS Scotland against these standards, and publishes the findings. The standards are based on the patient's journey as he or she moves through different parts of the health service. The standards set by NHS QIS are clear and measurable, based on appropriate evidence, and written to take into account other recognised standards and clinical guidelines. The way in which standards are developed is a key element to the quality assurance process. The system developed by NHS QIS ensures that members of the public are involved, as lay representatives, throughout the drafting and piloting of the standards and the subsequent review of services throughout Scotland.

NHS Quality Improvement Scotland published Maternity Services Standards in March 2005 (NHS QIS 2005). As part of the development of these standards, a pilot review was carried out in NHS Highland. A number of rural issues were identified at this time and, where appropriate, these were incorporated into the final version. The final standards have been split into five broad areas covering Core Principles, Pre-conception and Very Early Pregnancy, Pregnancy, Childbirth and Postnatal and Parenthood. These standards apply across all maternity services in Scotland, both urban and rural, so how NHS Boards develop their services to meet the standards can vary widely. The more remote and rural services have to be flexible and use innovative solutions to address some of the more challenging standards. All Health Board areas will be assessed as to their compliance with these standards and a report produced detailing their success in achieving them.

When considering a review of services and possible changes to the way care is being provided as described above, it is important to consider what impact these changes would have on the ability to meet these best practice standards. However, it should always be remembered that there can be challenges in meeting these standards when applying them to a remote and rural setting.

SUMMARY

Throughout this chapter it is clear that remote and rural communities face particular challenges in terms of transport, access to services and sustainability of local communities. Equally, healthcare staff who are providing care in these areas have to contend with the differing roles within the wider rural maternity team, staff competence and confidence in clinical practice and issues around skills maintenance and training.

Is it possible to balance the wishes of local communities or individuals in terms of locally available, high quality services with the aim of those providing the services to ensure that they are safe and sustainable?

This chapter has shown that it is possible to identify the risks which are associated with providing maternity care in a remote and rural area. It is also possible to discuss these with the woman and her family in a way that is meaningful to them. Making an informed choice is about balancing the risks associated with any particular course of action. Risks have to be identified, assessed as to their level of tolerability and then steps taken to reduce those which have been accepted to their lowest level possible.

The provision of high quality information which is accurate and unbiased is an essential requirement to allow people to make informed choices about their health and their healthcare. Information about the risks associated with living in a remote and rural setting must be included when people are making choices about the care they receive.

References

AS/NZS (Australian Standard/New Zealand Standard) 2004 Risk management (AS/NZS 4360). Standards Australia

Clements RV 1995 Essentials of clinical risk management. In: Vincent C (ed) Clinical risk management. BMJ Publishing Group, London, p 335–349

DH 1993 Changing childbirth (The report of the Expert Maternity Group). HMSO, London

DH 2001 Reference guide to consent for examination or treatment. Department of Health, London

DH 2003 Introduction of the 2003 consultant contract (England) [Advance letter: AL(MD) 3/2003]. Department of Health, London

DH 2004 Better information, better choices, better health: Putting information at the centre of health. Department of Health, London

NHS QIS (NHS Quality Improvement Scotland) 2003 Online. Available: http://www.nhshealthquality.org

NHS QIS 2005 Maternity services standards. NHS QIS, Edinburgh

NPSA (National Patient Safety Agency) 2005 The first report of the National Reporting and Learning System and the Patient Safety Observatory. Building a memory: preventing harm, reducing risks and improving patient safety. NPSA, London

RCOG/RCM (Royal College of Obstetricians and Gynaecologists/Royal College of Midwives) 1999 Towards safer childbirth – minimum standards for the organisation of the labour ward. RCOG Press, London

RCOG 2001 Clinical Governance Advice No 2. Clinical risk management for obstetricians & gynaecologists. RCOG, London. Online. Available: http://www.rcog.org.uk/ index.asp?PageID=477

Scottish Executive 2001 Framework for maternity services in Scotland. Scottish Executive, Edinburgh

Scottish Office 1993 The provision of maternity services in Scotland: a policy review. Scottish Office Home and Health Department, Edinburgh

SEHD (Scottish Executive Health Department) 2002a Report of the Expert Group on Acute Maternity Services: Implementing a framework for maternity services in Scotland. SEHD, Edinburgh

SEHD 2002b Advisory Group to Review the Scottish Medical Workforce (the Temple Report). Future practice: proposals of an advisory group to review the Scottish medical workforce. SEHD, Edinburgh

SEHD 2004a Informing, engaging and consulting the public in developing health and community care policies and services. SEHD, Edinburgh

SEHD 2004b New consultant contract [NHS Circular: PCS(DD)2004/2]. SEHD, Edinburgh

SEHD 2005 National framework for service change in the NHS in Scotland (the Kerr Report). SEHD, Edinburgh

Chapter **8**

Risk and Normality in Maternity Care: Revisioning Risk for Normal Childbirth

Denis Walsh

INTRODUCTION

Childbirth could be said to be in crisis across the Western world. At the beginning of the 21st century when birth has never been safer, it is increasingly rare for women to negotiate a path through labour without technology and drugs. Research has revealed the diminishing capacity for primigravid women to birth physiologically. In one study (Downe et al 2001), only 17% made it through labour without interventions like epidurals and caesarean sections. Even in midwifery-led case where the focus is specifically on normal labour and birth, oxytocin to speed up labours is widely used and electronic fetal monitoring almost ubiquitous (Mead 2004). The vast majority of births occur in hospitals, attended by midwives and obstetricians, suggesting that women have lost faith in their own abilities to birth without this medical and professional infrastructure of support. Pervading this context of childbirth is the ubiquity of risk which many believe is feeding defensive and interventionist practices in maternity care (Bassett et al 2000, Saxell 2000).

This chapter explores the reasons for these trends and develops a critique of the risk discourse that, it is argued, is driving these changes in maternity services. Alternative viewpoints from sociologists, midwives and service users are discussed as a way of addressing the crisis in physiological birth. How the risk agenda can be transformed into an enabling mechanism is developed towards the end of the chapter.

THE RISK DISCOURSE

Risk appears all pervasive in contemporary society, despite unprecedented levels of prosperity and technological advance in the developed world. Critics have analysed this phenomenon, particularly in relation to healthcare, and have put forward a number of characteristics defining it. These herald significant departures from earlier societies' notions of risk and health.

McLaughlin (2001) tracks a movement from risk as a neutral concept to do with probabilities of an event happening or not happening, to risk framed only as negative or undesirable outcomes. In relation to health, this movement has taken on a particular potency, fed by discourses of evidence-based medicine and health education.

Evidence-based medicine purports to reduce or eliminate risks by the appropriate use of diagnostic aids and the implementation of effective treatments. Clarke & Proctor (2002), in their investigation of Nursing Development Units in the United Kingdom (UK), argue that these processes of diagnosis and treatment are predicated on quantitative research methods only, pushing more experiential, interpretive research approaches to the margins. In this way risk is constructed exclusively in clinical terms and its management becomes a scientific matter (McLaughlin 2001). Horlick-Jones (1998) suggests this strips risk assessment of its context specific embeddedness and reifies the process as objective and rational. Later it will be argued that context is essential in exploring the meaning of risk in maternity care.

Health education has shifted in emphasis away from governments and corporations providing healthy living conditions (provision of sanitation, reduction in pollutants) to the individual's responsibility for choosing healthy lifestyle options. Society is bombarded with data about the risks of certain behaviours to do with diet, exercise and sexual practices to name a few. The personalisation of these choices imparts a moral dimension to them so that the ignoring of risks is seen as irresponsible and reprehensible (Lipman 1999).

RISK DISCOURSE AND MATERNITY CARE

In a number of ways, maternity care is an exemplar of the effects of the risk discourse on health. Childbirth straddles an ambiguous divide between what some perceive as an essentially physiological event and others as a pathology waiting to happen.

These contrasting views have been conceptualised as emanating from differing models of care: a biomedical or technocratic model and a social model.

Walsh & Newburn (2002) proffer the characteristics of these models in Table 8.1.

The technocratic perspective sees birth as risky until proven otherwise. It desires to prevent the worst case scenario, regardless of the likelihood of that ever happening – an approach dubbed 'a maximum strategy' by Brady & Thompson (1981). This requires adopting a low threshold for intervening and a highly sceptical view of labour physiology. The model supervalues morbidity and mortality outcomes over all others, especially the psychosocial, and monitors outcomes by measuring what goes wrong. It also casts labouring women as patients, dependent on medical interventions to rescue them from deviations from the norm. Professional expertise and knowledge is highly sought after in this model and is considered authoritative, based on positivistic notions of objectivity, generalisability and certainty, all

Table 8.1 Models of maternity care

Technocratic	Social
body as machine	whole person
reductionism: powers, passages, passenger	integrate: physiology, psychosocial, spiritual
control and subjugate	respect and empower
expertise/objective	relational, subjective
environment peripheral	environment central
anticipate pathology	anticipate normality
technology as master	technology as servant
homogenisation	celebrate difference
evidence	intuition
safety	self-actualisation

of which are obtained through quantitative research designs.

Sociologists (e.g. Fahy 1998, Lauritzen & Sachs 2001) have typified these values as belonging to the techno-rational paradigm that views science as progressive and modern. Techno-rationalism not only determines what counts as knowledge but also supports an industrial model of productivity or work. Such a view endorses efficiency and bureaucracy as fundamental to work systems. Risk assessment becomes another tool to fine tune efficiency in labour care. Centralised provision for childbirth requires such a model and mimics assembly-line production (Perkins 2004). This mainstream industrial model of maternity care in effect processes women through the phases of care. The organisational imperative to move women in at one end and out at the other end of hospital birth results in acute time pressures. Later in this chapter the invisibility of this organisational imperative to the risk assessment process will be explored. Labours have to be completed within a certain time frame and, therefore, they are frequently accelerated if perceived to have fallen behind the clock.

Friedman's (1954) work on labour length pathologised long labours, associating them with uterine rupture, creating a clinical imperative for time restrictions. However, accelerating labour often leads to other interventions. This is the territory of iatrogenesis, highlighted over 25 years ago by Illich (1977). He warned of the dangers of iatrogenesis and childbirth's recent history demonstrates a good example. At the beginning of the 1970s, electronic fetal monitoring was introduced to labour wards with the promise of reducing the incidence of perinatal mortality and morbidity linked to birth asphyxia. No such reduction occurred but the price that was paid was dramatic increases in caesarean sections for fetal distress; in some cases rates went up by 150% (Thacker 1997). It was not until much later that randomised controlled trials demonstrated no advantage for this technology over intermittent auscultation of the fetal heart (Thacker et al 2004).

Scenarios described above, repeated time and time again across maternity hospitals in the Western world, encourage the development of a risk mindset in relation to labour and birth. Obstetrics is considered by risk assessors to be extremely vulnerable to litigation and is therefore a particular target of risk management strategies. This is because of the huge payouts by maternity units for victims of cerebral palsy if the units are found culpable. Risk management resonates with wider concerns in society about growing uncertainty and insecurity and, as already stated, reveals something of a paradox: we feel increasingly vulnerable to biological, environmental and technological developments, despite decreasing mortality and morbidity rates in Western cultures.

Manuals on the rationale for risk management and its operational mechanisms rarely explore the assumptions underlying it or its philosophical antecedents, all of which contribute seminally to what could be called a 'discourse of risk' (Crawford 2004). Crawford (2004: 507) develops his argument regarding a disjunction between the goal of health and the 'disordered experience of its attempted achievement' by identifying a number of characteristics in contemporary medical culture that contribute to a culture of fear. Some of these have strong resonance with current maternity care. Crawford writes of the growth in health education to assist individuals in their healthy lifestyle choices. As already mentioned, these focus on risks to personal health and amount to a 'pedagogy of danger'. Information to newly pregnant women can resemble this: guidance on food and beverages to eat and avoid, drugs to avoid, behaviours to change (smoking, stress-inducing), recommendations on safe places of birth (access to neonatal facilities, avoid home), early and regular contact with specialist maternity services (obstetricians). These reinforce the 'preciousness' of the pregnancy condition.

Crawford's second characteristic is the role of technologies in identifying risk factors and detecting early disease. This has spawned whole new categories of hidden pathology, predispositions and susceptibilities. Screening for fetal abnormality is a typical example. This has grown exponentially over the past 15 years on the back of increasing sophistication with ultrasound techniques. What began with early detection of neural tube defects has burgeoned into the identification of an apparently increasing number of genetic and/or hereditary conditions in utero. Unfortunately, in many cases diagnosis is provisional and throws up relative rather than absolute risks. This is the phenomenon of 'soft markers' (Getz & Kirkengen 2003) which can generate anxiety and ambivalence in women who have to make vexed decisions about the appropriate course of action (Filley 2000). Shickle & Chadwick (1994) dub this trend as 'screeningitis' – the emotional inflammation and angst caused by the practice of inexact testing.

Lauritzen & Sachs (2001) develop this idea as the problematisation of the normal where everyone starts out normal but is unable to secure their healthiness. Screening alerts them to the possibility of abnormality and the potential of a rare but theoretical risk of a future calamity. Everyone has a small chance of great misfortune and in effect become a 'not-yet-patient'. A cursory glance at maternity care notes reveals this potential. One UK maternity service lists over 60 risk factors for pregnancy in their history-taking page (Walsh 2003). Evidence exists of the impact that a label of 'at risk' has on individual women as Williams & Mackey's (1999) study of women treated for preterm labour shows. The reality is that risk does not remain a statistic. It is 'experienced' by an individual and may well contribute towards the shaping of her identity.

It is known that the identification of risk factors in pregnancy is an inexact science, as Campbell demonstrated (1999) in her review of booking criteria utilised by various maternity services for home birth and birth centres. There was little agreement between them, probably contributing to the postcode lottery of home birth provision throughout England and Wales (NCT 2004). Saxell's (2000) excellent review of risk scoring tools for pregnancy revealed their poor predictability, adding to the argument that risk assessment for childbirth is a flawed endeavour.

In Adelsward & Sachs' (1996) critique of the meaning of numeracy in epidemiology's identification of risk, they illustrate how population-based risks are translated inappropriately to individual risk by clinicians. An individual, identified as having risk factors, becomes a 'not yet ill' patient. Pregnancy already has its share of symptomless illness as mild pregnancy induced hypertension and intrauterine growth retardation illustrate. The power of numeracy is that it is perceived as objective and 'true' and it therefore powerfully inscribes potential illness on the individual. The nuances of the risk discourse also invite dichotomous thinking so a risk is either present or absent, leading to the implication that a risk-free state exists (Adelsward & Sachs 1996). This kind of woolly thinking reinforces the notion in maternity care that 'high-tech' hospitals are safer environments to give birth in because they can set in place measures to reduce the risk and rapidly treat its effects if they do occur.

CONTEXTUALISING RISK

These critiques of how risk is conceptualised, particularly in maternity services, show how it is presented as a rational process, objectively undertaken for the greater good. This normative reading of risk obscures underlying values and beliefs that align it with scientific rationalism and the health specialism's professional projects. Actually, the medical profession's response to both risk management and evidence-based healthcare was initially equivocal as they perceived them as undermining their clinical autonomy (Allen 2000, Harrison 1998). More recently, McLaughlin (2001) has argued that the medical profession has appropriated the evidence agenda and risk management as a way of re-cementing its authority. She suggests it has developed the roles of evidence interpreter for complex clinical problems, and of determining risk factors and at-risk behaviours for different clinical conditions. Both roles are attempts to rehabilitate their expert status, which had been buffeted by a number of high profile mistakes (Wilson 2002).

Clarke & Proctor (2002) and Lipman (1999) both argue that the current risk discourse orthodoxy is socially constructed and outline how health professionals retain the power to define and interpret it. Lippman's critique revolves around the use and abuse of 'choice' as a seminal characteristic of 21st-century healthcare. How choices are presented reflects how risk is understood. She demonstrates how options that define choice are professionally dictated and that it is hard for consumers to introduce alternatives to those offered. Levy's (1999) research goes even further by illustrating that even within the acceptable options, midwives still 'gently steer' women towards the option they are most comfortable with. For some women, the choices on offer are further circumscribed by their own paucity of resources, either to articulate their specific needs or to glean sufficient information from their carers to enable an informed choice to be made. Kirkham (2004) continues to problematise the choice mantra as currently operationalised in maternity services. Drawing on disparate examples, her contributors deconstruct choice to demonstrate that, in the main, it is empty rhetoric and a placebo for policy-makers and strategists. At worst, it carefully circumscribes maternity care options and actually restricts choice for many women.

Crawford (2004) makes the astute observation that the ritual of risk as realised in medical culture makes us fear the unlikely but be unconcerned about the truly dangerous. Though paradoxical, this observation has resonance with how choices around place of birth and style of care are made in current maternity services. The discussion leads to the heart of contextualising risk assessment. As Anderson (2004) insightfully argues, a number of known risks that operate on large labour wards are ignored by risk assessment procedures which focus exclusively on the woman's own clinical features, rather than organisational deficiencies. These may include:

- lack of continuity of care and continuous support by midwives
- inexperienced doctors at the start of their rotation
- absence of expertise during the summer holidays, weekend night shifts, bank holidays
- disagreements between midwife and obstetrician
- inadequate handovers because of fatigue or intimidation

She adds to these incidental factors like unsupportive birth partners, bullying staff and a blame culture in completing her particular risk assessment for birthing on busy labour wards. The effects of a blame culture had been previously stressed by Ball et al (2003) in their UK study, exploring why midwives leave the profession. They found evidence of horizontal violence where many midwives felt under constant surveillance and feared reprisal if they made any errors. Stafford (2001) went further by suggesting that there is a current generation of 'what if' or 'just in case' midwives whose practice posture is defensive, linking this development to the ubiquity of risk. Irony abounds here as risk management strategy overtly emphasises a 'no blame' culture as an objective.

Anderson's contribution underscores the centrality of context in undertaking risk analysis. If context is ignored, then its influences remain invisible though they may represent the 'truly dangerous' as opposed to the potential and rare risks associated with the woman's medical history. Wagner (2001) articulates why contextual structural risks may be missed by risk assessors. He writes of the 'fish can't see water' syndrome. If risk assessors are embedded within the organisation where assessments are undertaken then how the organisation functions becomes normative. In effect, they are blinded to Anderson's factors.

Finally, to complete the critique of the risk discourse from the literature, Flynn (2002) argues that a new 'managerialism' is facilitating a control agenda by government in modern healthcare. The new managerialism has been borrowed from the private sector and is a kind of 'soft bureaucracy', both post-Fordist (a movement away from centralised bureaucratic, hierarchical models of organisation) and neo-Taylorist (preoccupations with quantifying processes and outcomes of work). The former promotes devolution of responsibilities and accountabilities to local hospital level while the latter requires a variety of measurements to be routinely collected and a number of clinical and organisational targets to be met. In this way, there is created at local hospital level a self-regulated, self-disciplined ethos that essentially addresses a centrally-driven agenda but ascribes full accountability for delivering the targets to the locality. For risk management this means that all risk strategy processes are developed and applied locally but the agenda is set by external agencies like those running the Clinical Negligence Scheme for Trusts (CNST). This powerful body indemnifies hospitals for insurance claims and is able therefore to dictate a variety of organisational and clinical standards for the hospital to fulfil prior to contractual agreement on insurance premiums.

REVISIONING RISK IN NORMAL CHILDBIRTH

In attempting to sketch out an alternative approach to risk management in maternity services, the following discussion emanates from beliefs and values of a social model of care. Deliberations are therefore based on a salutogenic or 'wellness' perspective of pregnancy and childbirth (Downe & McCourt 2004). A guiding principle becomes not the avoidance of risk but the promotion of efficacy. A starting point can be what evidence-based medicine tells us about care that supports physiological birth. It is a peculiar irony that the same examination of evidence sources that have been used to identify sundry risks to childbirth can also inform as to what facilitates normal labour and birth. Even more startling is the fact that positivist research designs deliver this verdict, despite Clarke & Proctor's (2002) assertion of the limitation of evidence-based medicine when predicated solely on these methods.

Systematic reviews and other quantitative studies conclude that birthing units existing alongside conventional labour wards and as geographically separate facilities (free-standing) appear to reduce labour interventions in women deemed to be at low risk (Hodnett et al 2006a,

Walsh & Downe 2004). Contributing to this low rate of intervention is probably the philosophy of carers in this setting which views labour and birth through a lens of normality. This focus on normality may also contribute to lower intervention rates in women deemed at be at higher risk, as a Canadian study showed (Ontario Women's Health Council 2001). In addition, women using these facilities are highly satisfied with their care. Researchers stress the centrality of a 'birth as normal' philosophy in achieving these outcomes (Esposito 1999, Coyle et al 2001). Esposito tells a remarkable story of a New York birth centre in capturing the power of philosophy to effect outcome. The birth centre explicitly adopted an 'active birth' approach to care that affirmed women's ability to birth without technology and medical interventions. Many of the women who came to the centre had previous negative experience of medicalised birth but over the course of their pregnancy internalised a new vision. From a pessimistic disposition about the likelihood of experiencing a normal labour, they became expectant and positive and many went on to have very natural labours and births at the centre.

Alongside findings about the efficacy of birth centres, a substantial body of research has examined the style and type of care that contributes to non-interventionist, successful physiological birth. These findings emphasise the value of continuity of care (Hodnett 2005) of having a midwife as a lead carer (Homer et al 2001) and of continuous support during labour (Hodnett et al 2006b).

These characteristics of care echo what Nolan (2002), a childbirth educator, believes to be fundamental to a proactive approach to risk management in maternity care. Her work also uses as a starting point promoting efficacy as opposed to identifying and avoiding risk. Her approach more aptly focuses on what women say are important themes in care provision, rather than what the professionals have researched. These have been identified many times by maternity service surveys and evaluations as the 3 Cs – choice, control and continuity. UK government policy explicitly endorsed them (DH 1993) and continued to endorse them (DH 2004). Nolan urges us to build services around these themes as they actually represent a preventative strategy. If combined with structural change to embrace birth centres and home birth and the endorsement of a 'birth as normal' philosophy, then maternity services can create the conditions to realise efficacy.

An important adjunct to this refashioning of service priorities to address known benefits and efficacy of different models of care, is the explicit acknowledgement that the current large scale, all-purpose, industrial model of labour care is failing women who anticipate having normal labour and birth. The corollary of all the research findings is that this model predisposes women to intervention and the widespread use of labour and birth technologies. The model itself has become a risk to normal birth. Contextualising risk assessment inevitably leads to this conclusion, yet there is little evidence that this is acknowledged or influences risk decisions. In fact, the evidence points to the reverse. Birth centres, both integrated and free-standing, struggle to be established (Walsh & Downe 2004), continuity of care pilot schemes are discontinued (Walsh 2001) and continuous support in labour remains an elusive objective for many units due to staff shortages (Walsh 2002).

Contextualising risk assessment has other implications for maternity services, in regard to their relationships with the institutional infrastructure of hospitals – Health and Safety, Infection Control departments. These bodies have jurisdiction over clinical environments and appear to predicate their risk assessment decisions on a world view that endorses linearity, simplicity and certainty. This is a kind of 'one size fits all' approach. Objective principles of safe handling and infection control are simply transplanted into each new situation without engaging with the particular factors that define them. Downe & McCourt (2004) critique these foundations of positivist knowledge generation in maternity care and their arguments could equally apply here. There are again a number of anecdotal examples in maternity care where these external agencies have reduced options for women and negatively impacted on midwives'

philosophy of care. Frustrating the provision of water birth because of health and safety concerns about the mobility of women and infection control worries over the cleaning of pools is one example. Restricting the availability of birth room props to facilitate active birth and requiring certain kinds of birth room décor when midwives want to create an ambience of home are other examples. But what of the risks of re-installing a more clinical and less homely environment when birth centres have the reverse as an explicit objective?

RISK AND SAFETY IN A BIRTH CENTRE

A recent ethnography of a free-standing birth centre in the UK revealed a contrasting language and meaning around the risk discourse (Walsh 2004). The inversion of the current orthodoxy around this topic could be said to be subversive as the following examples reveal.

BOOKING RATIONALE

There were a number of striking features in the women's accounts around reasons for booking at the birth centre. One of the most obvious was the absence of references to the technocratic model of childbirth. Women did not raise concerns about 'risk' and 'safety' at the birth centre, at least not in the way that these terms are usually understood. They did not comment on an absence of doctors, epidural provision, electronic fetal monitoring, facility for obstetric procedures like ventouse or caesarean deliveries, or an ambulance journey of at least 30 minutes if complications arose. Instead women focused on the social (family and friends' recommendations, proximity for visiting), the environment (calm, homely, small-scale, ease of parking, absence of busyness), and the personal (welcome, friendliness, helpfulness). In fact, their response to the technocratic model was negative when they had previous experiences of birth at larger consultant units.

It was clear that, for many, the first visit to the birth centre was very influential in their decisions to book there. In particular, the visit seemed to precipitate an immediate decision regarding the right place of birth for them. For many, this appeared an intuitive process that either simply felt right ('Yep – this is the sort of place') or could be visualised as the only appropriate place. As one woman said, 'I could picture myself at the Valley.' This response portrays the affective component of decision-making that is non-rational and non-scientific. It is immediate and 'right', rather than considered and weighed like probability-related decisions are. Sometimes idiosyncratic aspects of their lives influenced their considerations. The birth centre was seen as the best environment for a woman who was an insomniac. Another woman chose the centre because the nearest consultant unit was where her husband's mother had recently died of cancer.

All these examples serve to undermine the idea that evidence regarding the mortality and morbidity rates of different places of birth will be the dominant influence on women's decision-making.

NESTING INSTINCT

The study also revealed a shared preoccupation (midwives and women) with the birth environment. The midwives were continually honing the physical environment through regular make-overs to optimise it for birthing. Though this was clearly important for the women, an additional dimension to environment emerged from the data – women's concern for the emotional ambience of the birth setting. This was illustrated by one woman's experience of visiting the unit. She was greeted at the door by a staff member holding a baby and she concluded that this was a baby-friendly place. It seemed to her 'the most natural thing in the world to find in an environment where babies are born' though it is uncommon in large hospitals where there is active discouragement of carrying babies around because of health and safety concerns. Women in the study were seeking a birth ambience characterised by compassion, warmth, nurture and love.

The focus on environmental and emotional ambience is interpreted in the study as characteristic of the nesting instinct. Human nesting instinct appears to seek out the right emotional ambience for childbearing, which is as integral to establishing a protective, safe place for birth as are the immediate physical surrounds. The links with the previous discussion on choosing the appropriate place of birth are clear: the non-rational immediacy of decision-making when women visited the centre suggests an intuitive and rapid appraisal of emotional and environmental ambience. Similarly, it was the absence of the right emotional ambience in the other maternity units they visited (the more formal and depersonalised interactions with staff during their visits), together with their unsuitable physical environments that turned women against them.

Many of the women actually constructed meaning around the birth centre to redefine its purpose away from being a hospital or health service institution. Several women used the phrase 'it's not a hospital' and others suggested a number of alternatives – 'like home', 'my bedroom' and 'our living room', or 'like a bed and breakfast', 'like a hotel', even 'like a holiday camp' or 'a health farm'. These descriptions were attached to characteristics, sometimes juxtaposing their experience of a typical hospital with their experience of the birth centre. Clearly, their thinking was unrelated to the traditional understanding of the risk discourse of childbirth safety. In fact, their thinking inverts the risk discourse's logic of protection and safety by deliberately choosing a non-medical environment for birth. For the women, protection and safety appeared to mean reducing the risk of iatrogenesis associated in their minds with hospital birth.

These findings don't actually challenge the alignment of risk and safety for they seem to support an endorsement of the need for safety. It is the interpretation of what constitutes safety that is challenged here. Safety for these women had to do with their babies being protected rather than monitored, nurtured rather than managed and loved rather than cared for. For many, the traditional hospital was a threat to these aspirations, so much so that they took the radical step of deliberately redefining the facility away from the language of hospital and medical care.

It may be that if service users, as Nolan (2002) urges, were the main arbiters of a risk strategy for maternity services, then it would look very different from what is currently on offer. Along with the birth centre women in this study, they might rehabilitate the homely, the social and the interpersonal aspects of the childbirth event which have been largely dismantled by the technocratic and industrial approach. They might even change the process and outcome data so targeted at the moment on interventions like epidurals and morbidities like caesarean section to wellness markers like physiological labour, normal birth and personal empowerment.

CONCLUSION

Labour and birth care in the 21st century are in danger of being swamped by defensive practices emanating from an obsession with risk. The cost is in the rates of increasing childbirth interventions and in the emergence of tocophobia (fear of labour) as a psychological illness (Hofberg & Brockington 2000). There may also be long-term implications for future generations as research continues to link babies exposed to medicalised, traumatic births with destructive adult behaviours like suicide (Jacobson & Bygddeman 1998), eating disorders (Cnattingius et al 1999) and drug abuse (Nyberg et al 2000).

Now is the time to take stock and to reframe avoidance of risk with likelihood of efficacy and to begin to restore confidence in physiological birth before it is too late.

References

Adelsward V, Sachs L 1996 The meaning of 6.8: Numeracy and normality in health information talks. Social Science and Medicine 43(8): 1179–1187

Allen I 2000 Challenges in the health services: the professions. British Medical Journal 320: 1533–1535

Anderson T 2004 Conference presentation. The impact of the age of risk for antenatal education. NCT conference, Coventry, 13th March

Ball L, Curtis P, Kirkham M 2003 Why do midwives leave? Royal College of Midwives, London

Bassett K, Iyer N, Kazanjian A 2000 Defensive medicine during hospital obstetric care: a by-product of the technological age. Social Science and Medicine 51: 532–537

Brady H, Thompson J 1981 The maximum strategy in modern obstetrics. Journal of Family Practice 12(6): 997–999

Campbell R 1999 Review and assessment of selection criteria used when booking pregnant women at different places of birth. British Journal of Obstetrics and Gynaecology 106: 550–556

Clarke C, Proctor S 1999 Practice development: ambiguity in research and practice. Journal of Advanced Nursing 30(4): 975–982

Cnattingius S, Hultman C, Dahl M et al 1999 Very preterm birth, birth trauma, and the risk of anorexia nervosa among girls. Archive of General Psychiatry 56: 634–638

Coyle K, Hauck Y, Percival P et al 2001 Ongoing relationships with a personal focus: mothers' perceptions of birth centre versus hospital care. Midwifery 17: 182–193

Crawford R 2004 Risk ritual and the management of control and anxiety in medical culture. Health: An Interdisciplinary Journal for the Social Study of Health, Illness and Medicine 8(4): 505–528

DH 1993 Changing childbirth: report of the Expert Committee on Maternity Care. HMSO, London

DH 2004 The Children's National Service Framework. Online. Available: http://www.dh.gov.uk/PolicyAndGuidance/H ealthAndSocialCareTopics/ChildrenServices/Ch ildrenServicesInformation/fs/en

Downe S, McCourt C 2004 From being to becoming: reconstructing childbirth knowledges. In: Downe S (ed) Normal childbirth: evidence and debate. Churchill Livingstone, London

Downe S, McCormick C, Beech B 2001 Labour interventions associated with normal birth. British Journal of Midwifery 9(10): 602–606

Esposito N 1999 Marginalised women's comparisons of their hospital and free-standing birth centre experience: a contract of inner city birthing centres. Health Care for Women International 20(2): 111–126

Fahy K 1998. Being a midwife or doing midwifery. Australian Midwives College Journal 11(2): 11–16

Filley R 2000 Obstetric sonography: the best way to terrify a pregnant women. Journal of Ultrasound in Medicine 19: 1–5

Flynn R 2002 Clinical governance and governmentality. Health, Risk and Society 4(2): 155–173

Friedman E 1954 The graphic analysis of labour. American Journal of Obstetrics and Gynaecology 68: 1568–1575

Getz L, Kirkengen A 2003 Ultrasound screening in pregnancy: advancing technology, soft markers for fetal chromosomal aberrations and unacknowledged ethical dilemmas. Social Science and Medicine 56: 2045–2057

Harrison S 1998 The politics of evidence-based medicine in the United Kingdom. Policy and Politics 26(1): 15–31

Hodnett ED 2005 Continuity of caregivers during pregnancy and childbirth (Cochrane Review). In: The Cochrane Library, Issue 1, 2006. John Wiley, Chichester

Hodnett ED, Downe S, Edwards N et al 2006a Home-like versus conventional birth settings (Cochrane Review). In: The Cochrane Library, Issue 4, 2005. John Wiley, Chichester

Hodnett ED, Gates S, Hofmeyr GJ et al 2006b Continuous support for women during childbirth (Cochrane Review). In: The Cochrane Library, Issue 1, 2006. John Wiley, Chichester

Hofberg K, Brockington I 2000 Tokophobia: an unreasoning dread of childbirth: A series of 26 cases. British Journal of Psychiatry 176: 83–85

Homer C, Davis G, Brodie P et al 2001 Collaboration in maternity care: a randomised trial comparing community-based continuity of care with standard hospital care. British Journal of Obstetrics and Gynaecology 108: 16–22

Horlick-Jones T 1998 Meaning and contextualisation in risk assessment. Reliability Engineering and System Safety 59: 79–89

Illich I 1977 Limits to medicine: medical nemesis, the expropriation of health. Marian Boyers, London

Jacobson B, Bygddeman M 1998 Obstetric care and proneness of offspring to suicide as adults: a case control study. British Medical Journal 317: 1346–1349

Kirkham M 2004 Informed choice in maternity care. Macmillan, London

Lauritzen S, Sachs L 2001 Normality, risk and the future: implicit communication of threat in health surveillance. Sociology of Health and Illness 23(4): 497–516

Levy V 1999 Maintaining equilibrium: a grounded theory study of the processes involved when women make informed choices during pregnancy. Midwifery 15: 109–119

Lipman A 1999 Choice as a risk to women's health. Health, Risk and Society 1(3): 281–291

McLaughlin J 2001 EBM and risk: rhetorical resources in the articulation of professional identity. Journal of Management in Medicine 15(5): 352–363

Mead M 2004 Midwives' perspectives in 11 UK maternity units. In: Downe S (ed) Normal childbirth: evidence and debate. Churchill Livingstone, London

NCT (National Childbirth Trust) 2004 Call for more help on home births. Online. Available: http://news.bbc.co.uk/1/hi/health/4033051.stm

Nolan 2002 The consumer view. In: Wilson J, Symon A (eds) Clinical risk management in midwifery: the right to a perfect baby. Books for Midwives Press, Oxford, p 124–137

Nyberg K, Buka S, Lipsitt L 2000 Perinatal medication as a potential risk factor for adult drug abuse in a North American cohort. Epidemiology 11: 715–716

Ontario Women's Health Council 2001 Attaining and maintaining best practices in the use of caesarean sections. Online. Available: http://www.womenshealthcouncil.on.ca/English/page-1-361-1.html

Perkins B 2004 The medical delivery business: health reform, childbirth and the economic order. Rutgers University Press, London

Saxell L 2000 Risk: theoretical or actual. In: Page (ed) The new midwifery: science and sensitivity in practice. Churchill Livingstone, London

Shickle D, Chadwick R 1994 The ethics of screening: is 'screeningitis' an incurable disease? Journal of Medical Ethics 20: 12–18

Stafford S 2001 Is lack of autonomy a reason for leaving midwifery? The Practising Midwife 4(7): 46–47

Thacker S 1997 Lessons in technology diffusion: the electronic fetal monitoring experience. Birth 24(1): 58–60

Thacker S, Stroup D, Peterson H 2004 Continuous electronic fetal heart monitoring during labour (Cochrane Review). In: The Cochrane Library Issue 4, 2004. Update Software, Oxford

Wagner M 2001 Fish can't see water: the need to humanize birth. International Journal of Gynaecology and Obstetrics 75: S25–S37

Walsh D 2001 Birthwrite: continuity and caseload midwifery. British Journal of Midwifery 9 (11): 671

Walsh D 2002 Birthwrite: small is beautiful. British Journal of Midwifery 10(5): 272

Walsh D 2003 Birthwrite: maternity notes – a jaundiced account. British Journal of Midwifery 11(4): 268

Walsh D 2004 Becoming mother: an ethnography of a free-standing birth centre. PhD thesis (unpublished). University of Central Lancashire, Preston

Walsh D, Downe S 2004 Outcomes of free-standing, midwifery-led birth centres. Birth 31(3): 222–229

Walsh D, Newburn M 2002 Towards a social model of childbirth. Part 1. British Journal of Midwifery 10(8): 476–481

Williams S, Mackey M 1999 Women's experience of pre-term labour: a feminist critique. Health Care for Women International 20: 29–48

Wilson J 2002 Clinical risk modification: a collaborative approach to midwifery care. In: Wilson J, Symon A (eds) Clinical risk management in midwifery: the right to a perfect baby. Books for Midwives Press, Oxford, p 15–36

Chapter 9

Risk Discourse in the UK: An Obstetric Perspective

Pall Agustsson

INTRODUCTION

Risk management has had its place in clinical practice in the National Health Service (NHS) since its arrival in the 1950s, most often in an unstructured way that did not deliver the necessary improvements inpatient care and safety. Proactively pursuing structured risk management is a relatively new concept in the NHS, put in place to ensure the provision of safer care for patients. It follows the publication of several documents from the Department of Health pertaining to England and Wales over the past 5 years. Changes in clinical practice are necessary to achieve this goal and must, in addition to exercising risk management, take into account and accommodate choices in healthcare.

CHOICE AND CONSENT

It has become increasingly important for healthcare workers to appreciate and become proactive in practising risk management, especially as the provision of choice for patients has gained prominence on the agenda in the healthcare setting and is widely publicised. Patients are given a range of options and choices for their healthcare plans and are encouraged to express their preference. This is particularly important in the provision of maternity services where the majority of women are healthy and low risk at the outset of pregnancy. It seems therefore reasonable that where safe options are available women should be empowered to express their preferences. Pregnancy complications in low risk women do, however, frequently occur and it is therefore of paramount importance that both women, their partners and healthcare professionals are acutely aware that choices and risks coincide in all healthcare systems and are inextricably linked. How to make choices and decisions and at the same time limit risks is a major undertaking and a significant part of day-to-day working in clinical practice.

Over the past decade, patients' awareness of choices and informed consent has had an ever increasing role to play in decision-making and in the development of care plans. At the same time, healthcare workers have been forced to recognise and acknowledge the reality that clinical decisions in patient management can also be looked at as choices or options. They need to be aware that complex decision-making is often required and that patients need to be involved when decisions are made. Given the complexity of factors that impact on any individual decision it is inevitable that uncertainty in decision-making may arise on the part of the professional and that conflict may on occasion arise between the patient and the professional.

The importance of offering choice and gaining informed consent is a very prominent feature in most documents published recently by the Department of Health in the UK, the Royal College of Obstetricians and Gynaecologists and the Royal College of Midwives. But what informed consent really is, and what it entails, can be debatable. Can patients realistically give fully informed consent? To give informed consent implies a full understanding of what is being discussed. Can every patient after consultation and discussion about the medical care and treatment fully understand the information given in order to make a decision to give or withhold consent? Do patients really comprehend the extent of the consequences if risks that have been discussed do materialise? Patients today are more likely than in the past to challenge and disagree with the professional advice given, in spite of being advised about the risks

attached to the option they choose. It can therefore be a dilemma for professionals deciding how detailed the information provided should be, given the fine line between informing, advising and scaremongering. Fortunately, in most situations the likelihood of an adverse event occurring is low and most patients do not suffer adverse clinical incidents. The frequency of the adverse clinical incident is however not the only denominator. The severity of the potential outcome has additionally to be taken into consideration. Professionals have a responsibility to convey this information to women and to inform them about choices and risks. If an adverse clinical incident occurs, the question can arise concerning who carries the responsibility and who is accountable. Would the patient, for instance, be willing to accept responsibility having made a choice against professional advice? If not, should they be made to do so? During consultation and discussion it has to be made explicitly clear that both patients and professionals must accept that accountability and responsibility follow on from exercising choice and making decisions.

Adequate documentation of all consultations is vital as evidence of discussion having taken place. Case note review following adverse clinical incidents has shown poor documentation to be present all too frequently, and this in itself constitutes a major risk within maternity care, particularly if cases proceed to litigation.

THE 'NO ZERO RISK FACTOR'

It is essential that both healthcare providers and the public appreciate that in healthcare provision there is no 'zero risk' situation. At the same time, however, there are different perspectives from which this concept can be examined and managed. For instance, the approach in maternity care could be to consider that no event is normal except retrospectively and therefore to anticipate risks and make choices and plans accordingly. The other end of the spectrum is to manage pregnancy and childbirth as normal until abnormal signs appear. Alternatively, the probability factor can be employed, risk assessment carried out and a management plan made accordingly in agreement with the patient. All professionals have responsibility to patients, employers and their profession, but the risk management approach favoured may differ among the various professional groups, between individuals within the professions and between patients themselves. The medical view is possibly skewed towards abnormality and therefore expressed in a need to be proactive and to intervene early in spite of little evidence (or even an absence) of signs of abnormality. Midwives' training, on the other hand, places strongest emphasis on normality. However, within both professions individuals may have widely varying attitudes towards normality and its management.

Most patients when discussing care and outcome postnatally appear to be satisfied with a favourable outcome (i.e. a healthy mother and a healthy baby) regardless of whether it was achieved normally or by intervention. Dissatisfaction with care is often associated with poor communication and lack of explanation of the care provided, especially if an adverse event occurred or if labour and delivery did not meet the woman's expectations. A growing number of women, however, express strong views in the antenatal period about how pregnancy, labour and childbirth should be, and some have difficulty in accepting when these expectations are not met. They can therefore have a tendency subsequently to put the blame on healthcare professionals providing the care under these circumstances. Tension or conflict between the various healthcare professionals and women and their partners may therefore arise during attempts to find a mutually acceptable safe, low risk option. Due to the 'no zero risk factor' the service providers have to acknowledge that there are inherent risks present in maternity care and robust arrangements have to be in place to detect and manage these appropriately, and perhaps more significantly to manage unexpected or unanticipated events effectively.

RISK AND DECISION-MAKING IN MATERNITY CARE

When healthcare policies, protocols and guidelines are developed, providers of maternity care take into account what is the safest, most clinically effective and most acceptable care for the majority of the population concerned. These decisions have to be balanced by the constraints that the service must be cost effective and provided within the limits of available resources. The agreed policies put in place will therefore never be entirely risk free and it has to be recognised and accepted that there will be some trade-offs and that this will inevitably result in adverse clinical events occurring. The likelihood or frequency of events and the severity of their consequences must therefore be taken into consideration. One example to illustrate this is the consideration of induction of labour. Induction of labour is recommended between 10 and 14 days past 40 weeks' gestation based on the evidence that at 40 weeks the risk of stillbirth is 1 in 1000 and increases to 3 in 1000 at 42 weeks' gestation. No one would argue that the former is preferable to the latter. However, at the same time it must be recognised that induction of labour, especially in the first-time mother, is associated with a longer labour, higher use of regional analgesia for pain relief, operative delivery and their sequelae. The professional must convey all of this information to women and their partners in a way that allows the woman to understand what the implications are of consenting to or withholding consent for induction of labour.

Another illustration is the caesarean section rate. The caesarean section rate in most obstetric units in Britain is now over 20%, compared to 10% in the 1980s, and has increased steadily over the past two decades. This has not significantly decreased perinatal mortality over the same time period but there is some evidence that reduction in perinatal morbidity has been achieved. The government and relevant professional bodies are alarmed over this increase in rate, and want measures taken to reduce it. At the same time a significant factor in the increase of caesarean section is women's choice. Clinicians must then choose a path between satisfying official demands and women's choices, compliance with women's choice being in itself a recommendation from the government.

Professionals providing health or medical care often have differing views and approaches in how they administer and manage care. This is especially noticeable in the provision of maternity care. The aim of patients, midwives and medical professionals has the same end point, a physically and emotionally healthy, mother and baby, but the means to achieve this goal can take different routes.

It is ingrained in medical professionals during their training that they must become competent and confident in decision-making and be able to solve problems successfully. In the acute or emergency specialities such as maternity care, decisions often have to be made and acted upon rapidly. Frequently these decisions are irreversible and if the wrong decision is made or if things go wrong the consequences can be catastrophic resulting in a damaged or dead baby and traumatised mother. How can medical professionals make sure that the decision made is the most appropriate one, is the right one? It must also be appreciated that there is often more than one choice available and sometimes there is uncertainty regarding the right or the most appropriate choice. Additionally, there are clinical situations where there is no clear or obvious right answer. An example of this is in the management of extreme prematurity, to deliver or not, how and when. Consideration has to be given as to what the short-, medium- and long-term consequences are resulting from the decision made. How do professionals therefore reach a decision to manage a particular problem? Here we are guided by previous experience encountered in similar situations, by the most up-to-date current knowledge using best medical practice as a guide, and through discussions with colleagues working as a team. Protocols and guidelines to manage known or commonly occurring problems in the form of algorithms are now seen as mandatory in

maternity care, particularly in the labour ward, to ensure risk reduction and an appropriate management care plan. These are important tools to streamline management, make it consistent and aid medical and midwifery professionals to manage the clinical situation appropriately, but there will always be instances that don't fit the scenario comfortably.

Midwives too recognise that maternity care has risks associated with it and they too follow protocols and guidelines and use algorithms as an aid to decision-making. The midwife's perspective, however, is more focused on an anticipated normality for pregnancy, labour and delivery. There is greater expectation on their part that the woman's progress will be uncomplicated. Amongst other things, previous work experience may influence the perception of risks. Those who have worked in general practitioner (GP)- or midwife-led units are more likely to have supported women through normal labours and births and therefore have confidence that for the majority of women there is a need for support and little else, unless there is evidence of a complication arising. Their energies go into supporting normality and the early detection and transfer of women who develop complications with clear and concise protocols in place to facilitate and ensure safe practice. Midwives who have worked mainly in consultant-led maternity units, frequently with intensive feto-maternal monitoring and surveillance, are more likely to perform 'routine' assessments/ investigations, partly due to being influenced by medically-driven protocols and partly, it could be surmised, from their experience that a large proportion of the women for whom they provide care do suffer complications and require medical intervention. Their energies are more focused on the efficient provision of such interventions. There is some evidence that midwives from consultant-led units are reluctant to work in midwife-led units as they perceive the risk of complications and associated poor outcomes as being too high. Community midwives attached to the same consultant-led units are more likely to opt to work in a midwife-led unit, presumably because their experience of attendance at home births mirrors that of the midwives in GP- or midwife-led units. A major factor that will influence the risk-taking behaviour of midwifery and medical professionals as well as patients is the level of risks that is in general acceptable to them – some being risk averse, others being risk takers.

As midwives now provide total care to a large number of women, medical professionals can find themselves meeting a woman for the first time when she is at a point in her maternity care where significant decisions and changes must be made to her previously low risk care plan. Little or no discussion may have taken place before about potential medical interventions. This may lead to conflicts, especially as no relationship and trust has previously been established between the woman and the medical professional. Public expectations have steadily increased over the past decade and are often seen by healthcare professionals as unrealistic, especially as the occurrence of adverse clinical incidents is deemed unacceptable. Generally speaking, the public response is that someone is to blame and that someone has to pay. Patients are influenced by a multitude of factors, including ethnic background and cultural values, their own previous experience and that of friends and relatives. The media, including the internet, are now responsible for providing a huge amount of information, evidence based or otherwise, relating to pregnancy and childbirth. This leads women and their partners to form expectations about what pregnancy and childbirth should be like. Depending on the information at hand and individual circumstances, these expectations are not always realistic and can sometimes be impossible to achieve. When choice is being offered an assumption is being made that all patients have the capability to make sense of the large amount of information and often technical data that are being provided to them. Another assumption frequently made is that patients always want and know how to make choices. Not everyone is used to making conscious choices and a significant number of people are comfortable with and often prefer other people making choices

for them. It can be a very complex and time-consuming process for healthcare professionals to determine each patient's position in regard to this.

The UK government currently hugely supports normality in pregnancy and childbirth and this is strongly demanded and promoted by various women's groups such as the Association for Improvements in the Maternity Services (AIMS). Interestingly, however, some very pertinent government documents relating to maternity care – for example, the Framework for Maternity Services in Scotland (Scottish Executive 2001) – are very much focused on risks and safety. Normality or risk-free pregnancy and childbirth get very little mention.

Promotion of community-based midwifery-led care for low risk women, support of Community Midwives' Units and the development of 'normality' courses for midwives is indirect evidence of support for normality. The UK government at the same time realises the risk involved in maternity care and places strong emphasis on risk assessment and management.

RISK MANAGEMENT

In order to support normality and choices, minimise risks and learn from adverse events, an efficient and effective risk management is a prerequisite and is paramount in trying to ensure the highest standard of patient care and safety. Risk Evaluation Management needs to be an integral and essential part of the day-to-day working in clinical practice. This is supported by the Clinical Governance concept in the NHS. The publication of *A first class service: quality in the new NHS* (DH 1998a), followed by *The new NHS: modern, dependable* (DH 1998b) and *A plan for investment – a plan for reform* (DH 2000) laid down the foundation for active risk management within the NHS. The Clinical Governance structure is now, several years later, well embedded within the NHS with risk management playing a major part. Specific guidance pertaining to risk management issues that helps organisations to facilitate and structure effective and efficient risk management systems comes from various sources: government bodies, National Health Organisations, the medical, midwifery and nursing Royal Colleges, and the General Medical Council.

NHS trusts have a statutory and legal obligation to practise Clinical Governance and risk management within the organisation. In order for this process to be effective the risk management concept and its practice must reach beyond board and trust level, and robust risk management systems need to be in place and actively practised within each hospital clinical area.

Individuals clearly identified as responsible for the overall organisation and management of the risk management activity need to be in place. In high risk clinical areas a dedicated risk manager with no other contractual obligations needs to be in position in order to effectively manage risks and facilitate change. To achieve effective risk management, adverse clinical incidents need to be documented, reported, and investigated and the outcome managed appropriately with specific recommendations towards change in practice where necessary. It is therefore imperative that all the healthcare workers are motivated to participate in the process.

The Clinical Governance structure promotes openness, transparency and a blame-free culture in relation to adverse incidents. This is a different and novel approach from the past where blame, retributions and disciplinary actions were the norm. Cultural change is therefore required both from the management and the clinical side to facilitate successful reporting by staff involved in adverse clinical incidents, because if these are not reported the system fails. Fear of blame and retribution is, however, only one factor in under- or non-reporting. Well-defined adverse clinical incident lists need to be introduced and promoted and a user-friendly reporting system has to be in place to allow easy access to the risk management system. Adequate training in the use of the system, support and feedback are a prerequisite to successful reporting. Staff perceptions that reporting adverse clinical incidents makes a change and improves patient management and care are essential. In order to achieve this goal, dedicated commitment to active risk management at all levels in the health service is essential to facilitate and implement the necessary changes in practice.

RISK MANAGEMENT IN MATERNITY CARE

Pregnancy and childbirth are not diseases and it is appropriate that where possible they should be considered natural and normal to human existence and managed accordingly. This has, however, to be balanced against the possible risks. Maternity care is a difficult area to manage where risks and choices are concerned given the fact that obstetrics is a high risk clinical area where a significant proportion of complaints originate. Obstetrics has one of the highest litigation rates in medical practice with the highest cost and expense from medical claims and litigation. Currently, there is an ever increasing demand to de-medicalise maternity care. At the same time, human pregnancy and parturition are associated with significant risks. Adverse events, if they occur, are often irreversible, and may result in a damaged or dead baby and maternal death. We only have to look to parts of Africa and the Far East where the standard of maternity care is poor and maternal and infant death are a daily occurrence. Maternal and fetal mortality have decreased significantly in Britain over the past 50 years but deaths still occur. In most areas in Britain the stillbirth rate is fairly constant, around 5 per 1000 births, and has not seen a significant reduction over the past 10–15 years. Maternal mortality has also remained constant over the same time period. This has been partly achieved by proactive medical management of pregnancy and childbirth and as importantly by the improved general health of the population. Mortality is, however, only one measure but it can be easily quantified, morbidity on the other hand which is equally important is more difficult to assess and quantify.

Healthcare professionals all agree upon the low-key approach in managing maternity care but professionals cannot be complacent. Demedicalisation must be planned, controlled and monitored. Adequate training of midwives as the main or sole caregiver during low risk pregnancy is essential with a well structured pregnancy plan in place, giving clear pathways to follow if pregnancy complications or concerns arise. At present this presents difficulty in satisfying all stakeholders. The main and principal aim of risk management is to ensure the highest standard of patient safety and care. Achieving this aim will result in a reduction in the number of complaints and medical negligence claims and litigation, allowing valuable resources to stay within the healthcare system and utilised to achieve improved patients' care.

References

DH 1998a A first class service: quality in the new NHS. HMSO, London

DH 1998b The new NHS: modern, dependable. HMSO, London

DH 2000 A plan for investment – a plan for reform. HMSO, London

Scottish Executive 2001 Framework for maternity services in Scotland. Scottish Executive, Edinburgh

Chapter **10**

Conjuring Choice While Subverting Autonomy: Medical Technocracy and Home Birth in Ireland

Marie O'Connor

CONTEXT

IRISH MATERNITY CARE

Healthcare in Ireland is currently undergoing a period of cataclysmic 'reform', driven in part by the neo-liberal ideology of health for profit. Health services, hitherto regionalised, have recently been brought under a single authority. Almost 62 000 women give birth – under obstetric 'supervision' – in the country's 22 maternity facilities. Eleven of these are scheduled to close. The services are hypermedicalised: half of all first-time mothers give birth by caesarean section, vacuum extraction or forceps delivery (Bonham 2005: 111).

Choices in Irish maternity care are few. Community services are minimal: there are no free-standing birth centres, no birth houses. Since the mid-1970s, when nursing homes offering such facilities closed, more and more births have taken place in ever-larger hospitals and obstetric units (Bonham 2005: 67).

A SNAPSHOT OF HOME BIRTH

Home was the place of birth until the middle of the 20th century. At that time, general practitioner referral or 'urgent necessity' was a prerequisite for hospital 'confinement' (McQuillan 1994: 9). The 1970 Health Act gave women a legal entitlement to home birth services from the State. By the 1980s, however, home birth had become a vestigial part of a service that was based on centralisation, not localisation, on obstetrics, not midwifery, on institutionalisation, not home. Today, home birth is in jeopardy, mainly due to a concerted campaign to eliminate self-employed midwives.

As in Britain, the model for midwifery in Ireland is one of employment. Less than 0.75% of practising midwives work as independent practitioners, compared with 1.5% of midwives in Britain (European Workgroup of Independent Midwives 2000: 16). In Ireland, however, self-employed midwives work against a background of hostility from both medical consultants and general practitioners, non-cooperation from maternity hospitals and obstructionism from health authorities.

Demand for home birth services outstrips supply. While only 0.4% of births take place at home by choice (Bonham 2005: 1), a national survey (Wiley & Merriman 1997: 98) found that 14% of hospital birth mothers would have liked to give birth at home. Home birth is increasingly reserved for independent-minded, higher income women who succeed in sourcing one of the 14[1] (Home Birth Association: 2005) midwives in independent practice: some 216 mothers did so in 2000. From 1990 to 1999, the number of births attended by independent midwives rose by 59% (Cullen 2002: 1). These practitioners work mainly in the east and south of the country: all run specialist home birth practices. Hospital midwives provide skeletal home birth services in south Dublin.

THE RISE OF OBSTETRICS AND THE DECLINE OF MIDWIFERY

Why are Irish maternity services so unresponsive to women's wishes? The growth of private healthcare, the development of obstetrics, the invention of 'active management' and the consequent decline of midwifery, all – mediated by gender (O'Connor 2001a, Witz

1992) and/or economics – have played a significant role in shaping the services for birth.

In the past half-century or so, childbirth has changed from being a domestic event under the control of women (see Kane 1978) to being a medical procedure in institutions under the management of men. Since the beginning of the 1980s, women have increasingly challenged this hegemony. Public conflict between women and obstetrics has increased markedly in the past decade, particularly in Dublin. The dispute in Ireland, as elsewhere (see Pfeufer Kahn 1995, Wertz & Wertz 1977, Williams 1997) is a gendered one: 83% of consultant obstetricians in Ireland are male (Comhairle na nOspidéal (The Hospitals' Council) 2001: 22), as are 70% of general practitioners (Irish College of General Practitioners 1997: 14). Midwifery, in contrast, is over 99% female.

Private care also plays a significant role: over 50% of the population now hold private health insurance. Hospital doctors appointed to the coveted public post of 'consultant' are entitled to practise medicine privately, both on and off the site of their employment: the State gives them access, free of charge, to public facilities, including midwifery and medical time. Hospital midwives care for all obstetric 'patients', public and private.

Although all pregnant women are legally entitled to public services free of charge, many opt for private care. The market for private obstetrics is worth at least €49m annually; this is divided among the country's 104 obstetricians (www.comh-n-nosp.ie/pdf.ConsultantStaff 2005.pdf). Dublin doctors earn an estimated €503 000 on average annually from private maternity fees. Outside Dublin, where births are less centralised, revenues tend to be slightly lower, averaging €447 000 per head annually (see Endnote). These incomes are further boosted by public salaries (ranging from €125 to €150 000) and private gynaecological fees.

If Irish maternity care has a defining characteristic, it is 'active management'. Implemented at the National Maternity Hospital in 1963, the system was, and is, a blueprint standardising the medicalisation of first births (O'Connor 2001a). One of its stated objectives

---

[1] The newsletter lists 15 'independent domiciliary' midwives; the correct number is 14, however, as one of those listed is a hospital employee.

was to replace the old 'static' (midwifery) approach by a new 'dynamic' regime that gave obstetricians a managerial role in the labour ward (O'Driscoll et al 1993: 16). Active management redefined hospital midwives as (obstetric) nurses, stripping them of their autonomy; within this rigidly hierarchical system, independent midwifery, based as it was on physiological birth in non-institutional settings, could be seen as a deviation from the norm active management sought to create, that of institutionalised, medicalised birth.

Irish midwifery was regulated by the London-based Central Midwives' Board until 1950, when midwifery in Ireland was colonised by nursing. The Nurses' Act (1950) subsumed midwifery into nursing, setting up a single regulator for both professions, An Bord Altranais (The Nursing Board) (Commission on Nursing 1998: 42), which continues to this day. Midwives lost their title in 1985, with the passing of The Nurses' Act, which made it legal to refer to a midwife as a 'nurse'. Today, stifled by more than 40 years of nursing rule (and active management), the future of midwifery must be in doubt. While the number of registered midwives is around 12 000, only 2400 (16%) work in midwifery, some part-time (M Higgins, personal communication, 2004).

THE CONSTRUCTION OF RISK

As birth moved into hospital, its vicissitudes became institutionalised within a growing body of self-referencing medical knowledge. With the proliferation of a new medical specialty which claimed responsibility for the outcome of birth, danger was transformed into biomedically constructed notions of risk (Cartwright & Thomas 2001: 218). The language of risk reinforced the illusion of its elimination through management.

Gender additionally informed the view. Irish obstetrics developed a theory of 'female incompetence' (Murphy-Lawless 1998: 29-30) in the 18th century: this was 'the lynchpin used to justify obstetric control' (Murphy-Lawless 1989: 45). The obstetric view of risk also derives from

its view of itself; obstetrics initially saw itself as a mechanic repairing the-body-as-machine; then, later, after World War II, obstetrics viewed itself as a technocrat, managing the-body-as-system (Arney 1982: 8). Underlying these ideas was a 17th-century notion, the Cartesian belief that mind and body are separate and function independently of each other (O'Connor 1995: 250).

As medicine continued its slow but unrelenting colonisation of the female body in childbirth, the concept of risk changed profoundly. The mapping of the fetus enabled new frontiers to be opened up, bringing new dimensions of risk under the clinical gaze. From 1950 onwards, doctors began to treat the fetus as a second patient, finding in the child a way 'to blunt the critical edge of women's concerns about the way obstetricians treated them' (Arney 1982: 136).

Half a century later, fetal rights have been enshrined in law in many countries. Ireland amended its Constitution in 1983 to give the fetus a right to life equal to that of its mother (Tomkin & Hanafin 1995: 182). There is now a perception on the part of some obstetricians (and others) that legal proceedings to protect the fetus, authorising the non-consensual medical treatment of pregnant women, may succeed before the courts. Legal practitioners in Ireland, however, disagree (M Forde, personal communication, 2004).

From being a clinical assessment of an individual woman, risk has now become an all-encompassing, statistical miasma. Active management defined all women as being at risk, dissolving the boundaries between normal and abnormal birth and labeling healthy women with textbook pregnancies 'low risk'. New obstetric 'risks' were constructed, through the imposition of newly-created medical 'norms'. Time management in the labour ward, for example, a central feature of active management, required a woman's cervix to dilate at the rate of 1 cm per hour: risk then lay in deviation from that notional norm. Today, 'failure to progress', thus defined, is frequently listed as a risk requiring the transfer of a home birth mother to hospital during labour.

Active management institutionalised the domination of midwifery by obstetrics. The hospital midwife was seen as a member of the obstetric hierarchy, a 'mini-doc' reporting directly to the senior obstetric registrar (O'Driscoll et al 1993: 97). Within this perspective, the midwife who did not report to a doctor, or who did not practise according to medical rules, was suspect, as the Kelly Case (discussed below) demonstrated.

Active management, moreover, exhorted consultant obstetricians to openly declare 'full acceptance of responsibility for the outcome [of birth]', including 'mishaps' (O'Driscoll et al 1993: 96-97). But with responsibility came liability: mishaps led to malpractice suits. The wave of litigation that broke in the United States in the mid-1970s reached Ireland a decade later when the parents of a quadriplegic child succeeded in their action (*Dunne* v. *National Maternity Hospital* [1989]) (Tomkin & Hanafin 1995: 73). Litigation paranoia now permeates the services: the prospective bill for past liabilities, known and incurred by Irish obstetricians, is reported to be €400 m (Donnellan 2004).

SCHEDULING THE RISKS

However, the medical preoccupation with risk preceded the rise in malpractice cases. The development of computer technology permitted large-scale data analysis to be carried out, enabling medical risk to be presented as a 'scientific' construct. In Britain, surveys such as those done by the British Birthday Trust permitted doctors to devise new management strategies, such as risk scoring systems, to identify the fetus at risk. Protocols designed to reduce the uncertainty of childbirth followed, even where data supporting them did not exist (Cartwright & Thomas 2001: 218). While all attempts at standardising such systems failed, they advanced the obstetric project of 'integration'. Just as the British Obstetrical Society had done in 1825 (Park 2005), obstetricians now claimed midwifery as a medical specialty, albeit at a lower level of expertise: risk scoring systems were, and are, used to allocate women to different levels within the hierarchy. These rules

were seen to protect doctors against litigation, while at the same time enabling obstetrics to restrict midwives' services to women defined by doctors as 'low risk'.

Such strategies copper-fastened the medical control over midwifery practice, enshrined in law in Britain in 1902 (Park 2005).

Being small of stature, for example, rendered a woman suspect for home birth. In a recent High Court case in Dublin, a maternal height of less than 152 cm (Glan Hafren NHS Trust Midwifery-Led Care Protocol, undated) was included in a list of 'obstetric risk factors' submitted to the court (*Nevin-Maguire and Maguire* v. *South-Eastern Health Board* [1999] JR 346). Being unmarried was another British Birthday Trust disqualifier for midwifery-based care in the home (Chamberlain et al 1978). Now, 50 years later, home birth criteria continue to incorporate ill-defined, catch-all social factors, such as 'lack of family support' (see Brenner 2001, Appendix 2), which serve as tools to exclude women from home birth.

HOME BIRTH VIEW OF RISK

In Ireland, as in other countries, the home birth movement is grounded in feminism and complementary health (O'Connor 1995). Women choosing home birth often believe – frequently on the basis of personal experience – that hospital birth carries significant risks: they view home as a safer environment, particularly for the baby.

There is a wealth of evidence to support the view that hospital maternity care may not be particularly safe. Ireland's perinatal mortality rates are among the highest in the European Union (Bonham 2005: 15). In 2000 (the most recent year for which published perinatal data are available), perinatal mortality rates rose by 7.3% (Bonham 2005: 1). Hospital-acquired infections pose significant problems: a European study carried out in 1999 found a national methicillin-resistant *Staphylococcus aureus* (MRSA) rate of 39% (Department of Health and Children 2000: 32).

Women who choose home birth in Ireland are, in most cases, making a highly conscious choice in maternity care: home birth attitudes, values and beliefs tend to be similar to those found in other countries. Influenced by writers such as Sheila Kitzinger, such mothers also read home birth studies, particularly those published in Britain or Ireland (O'Connell & Cronin 2002, O'Connor 1995).

A national survey of intentional home birth in Ireland found that two out of every three women subscribed to 'natural childbirth', a belief system shared by home birth mothers everywhere (O'Connor 1995: 236). Most respondents believed that birth is safer in an environment where labour will not be actively managed. Women saw pregnancy and birth as 'natural', refusing to accept the medical idea that every birth is inherently pathological. Some saw the management of labour in hospital as authoritarian and repressive. Declining to accept the patient role with its consequent loss of autonomy, these women refused to accept the dualism – and the pathology – inherent in the two-patient model of childbirth. Natural childbirth was seen as the optimal way of ensuring the safety of mother and child. Home birth mothers who believed in non-intervention were not haunted by the spectre – often invoked by doctors – of the newborn baby who does not breathe: they believed that, at home, such babies are very rare, because of the way midwives manage birth. Women occasionally focused on specific risks: distance from their home to the nearest maternity unit was a consideration for some, while women who tended to have fast labours believed that home birth offered a safer solution than the alternative: an unattended roadside birth.

Theirs was a social, holistic model rooted in unity, the unity of mother and child, of mind and body (see also Davis-Floyd 1992, Katz Rothman 1982). Women who thought that mind and body were interdependent believed that the baby's physical safety depended, to a degree, on their own emotional wellbeing. They felt their labours would be easier if they were relaxed and confident. Home was seen to offer freedom from anxiety and the security of knowing their midwife. Within the group, women's view of

risk was buttressed by the certainty that, at home, medical interventions, which they generally perceived as risky, would not be imposed on them against their wishes. In their accounts, issues of autonomy intertwined with those of safety: home, unlike hospital, was perceived as offering both.

RESOLVING TENSIONS BETWEEN WOMEN AND DOCTORS

Tensions between women's views and medical perspectives continue: their resolution is nowhere in sight. Parliament, government and courts have combined to enact and enforce medical power over the services for birth. The State continues to uphold a system of maternity care based on obstetrics, enforcing it, where necessary, against parents' wishes.

BUILDING MEDICAL MONOPOLY

In Ireland, as in other countries, the medical profession has used its considerable power to carve out a monopoly position for itself. Medicine has succeeded in enlisting the full powers of the State in this project. In 1976, medical consultants claimed that birth was safer in maternity units staffed by themselves (Comhairle na nOspidéal 1976). No evidence was cited for this claim; today, Irish maternity care policy, unhindered by the weight of research on the safety of midwifery-based care, continues to promulgate this article of faith.

Ireland's scheme for community maternity services (known as the 'Mother and Child' scheme) is strongly reminiscent of Britain's system of 'combined care'. The system is presented as a scheme for medical services (McQuillan 1994: 9-11), combining general practitioner monopoly in the community with obstetric monopoly in hospital. The text barely acknowledges that community services may also be provided by midwives.

Legal, regulatory and other barriers to midwifery practice abound. As in other countries, midwives are legally restricted from exercising even limited prescribing powers. Suppliers, additionally, decline to supply: health authorities, for instance, refuse to supply midwives with home birth kits given free of charge to general practitioners (none of whom have attended home births for a decade or more).

MAINTAINING MEDICAL CONTROL

Since the 1960s, when the demand for home birth was articulated by women whose healthcare systems no longer offered this possibility, one of the overriding problems for obstetrics has been: how to maintain medical control over maternity services. In recent years, the hospital has been increasingly seen as the hub of service provision in the community, with hospital midwives, as in Denmark, providing 'integrated' home birth services under medical supervision. Primary care plays no discernible role in this model, nor do independent midwives (Condon, unpublished, 2000, Porter 2000).

The boundaries around clinical midwifery practice are drawn by multidisciplinary 'consensus' groups, which, like the 1902 Central Midwives Board of England and Wales (Park 2005), tend, invariably, to be medically dominated. The setting up of these groups, locally, nationally and internationally, has provided a modern solution to the age-old medical problem of how to retain power in modern healthcare systems while legitimising its exercise by giving it an appearance of democracy. In Ireland, multidisciplinary consensus groups have been intermittently established to 'review' maternity services. Such groups have recently been shown to cloak an increasingly authoritarian and repressive approach to policy-making.

The first review of the Mother and Child scheme took place in 1980; the largely medical group reiterated the theological belief that all women should be placed under obstetric management in hospital. In 1993, the Irish Medical Organisation secured a further review of the scheme with a view to replacing home birth services ('childbirth is no longer the major item it used to be for doctors') with more lucrative items, such as cervical screening and (postnatal) family planning (see Irish Independent 1992).

The concept of risk in these and other reports was amorphous and ill-defined, to be inferred from half a paragraph of unsubstantiated belief statements and policy pronouncements (McQuillan 1994: 18). Instead of facts, the largely medical committee cited opinions, invoking the stances of medical bodies to support its pro-hospitalisation policy. The oft-repeated obstetric view, that consultant-managed units offer the 'safest environment for deliveries', was reiterated: this policy, the group claimed, was 'responsible for the marked decrease in the level of maternal, perinatal and infant mortality'. No evidence was adduced in support of this rather sweeping assertion.

To contain what was now seen as a rising demand from women for greater control over birth, the McQuillan Group recommended the piloting of hospital domino and at-home-in-hospital schemes, stymieing the development of home birth services while appearing to respond to women's demands for such care. Hospital midwives, under medical direction, were to cater for that 'small number of women, who regardless of policy or professional advice, would insist on having a home birth' (McQuillan 1994: 23).

LEGAL, REGULATORY AND OTHER STRATEGIES

In the 1950s, general practitioners often succeeded in enlisting the Nursing Board in their efforts to restrict midwifery practitioners. Half a century later, a similar strategy was employed by the then Master[2] of the National Maternity Hospital, Peter Boylan, who lodged a complaint against independent midwife Anne Kelly in 1996. Without investigating his allegations, the Nursing Board took out a High Court injunction against Ms Kelly to prevent her from practising, following this with disciplinary proceedings. The home birth midwife was charged with exposing mother and baby to 'undue and serious risk', by allowing her client to labour at

---

[2] 'Master' is a 17th-century title, still used by Dublin maternity hospital obstetric chief executives.

home for a period of time well in excess of active management norms. Professional power was the issue; the alleged risk did not materialise; mother and child were well after the birth and the obstetrician took the complaint against the woman's wishes.

The fitness to practise case buttressed itself by reference to a National Maternity Hospital rule, which mandates hospital transfer in home birth if the baby shows signs of having had a bowel movement, during labour or prior to it. Whether or not the midwife should have transferred her client to obstetric care at the sight of meconium became the central issue. A senior hospital midwife told the fitness to practise inquiry that independent midwifery practice should be governed by National Maternity Hospital rules. But the evidence for the meconium 'guideline' failed to convince the committee; and, after a 4-year legal juggernaut, the midwife won her case on both the judicial and disciplinary fronts. By then, in its efforts to make midwifery subservient to medicine, the Nursing Board had spent an estimated €2 m on legal fees (C MacGeehin, personal communication, 2006).

Three months after the initial complaint against Anne Kelly, controlling the boundaries around midwifery practice had become an urgent necessity for obstetrics. In January 1997, health boards appointed an 'expert' group on home birth: service users were not represented. Repeating the mantra that consultant-staffed units were 'safest', the group recommended national standards incorporating rules for, among other things, the transfer, during labour, of home birth mothers.

Regional health authority pilot schemes soon followed. Two proposed that hospital midwives should provide midwifery services, including home birth, free of charge to women approved by doctors for such services. These mainly domino[3] schemes were under obstetric management. One such scheme resulted in a

hospital home birth rate of under 0.4%: it catered for less than 4% of patients, of whom 10% had a home birth (Brenner 2001: 12). The third scheme was community-based: in Cork, independent midwives were contracted by the local health authority – as provided for by the 1970 Act – to provide home birth services to selected women. Faced with evidence of its success, Cork obstetricians refused to cooperate with the midwives, citing their 'independence' as an insurmountable difficulty (Brenner 2004: 10).

Risk scheduling was central to these schemes. But while the schedules were promoted as 'scientific', they did not necessarily agree as to what constituted a risk. In Dublin, the project specified a maximum of 5 miles from the mother's residence to the hospital; while in Cork, a limit of 40 miles from the client's home to the midwife's residence was the criterion. One feature common to most schedules, however, was meconium. An established indication for in-labour transfer in home birth (see, for example, Obstetric Working Group, National Health Insurance Board of the Netherlands 2000: 21), meconium's status as an indicator of fetal distress in the mature baby remains unproven.

As in Britain, these schedules represented a medicalisation of home birth, influenced, as they were, by the culture of active management. Women's 'failure to progress' in the first stage of labour was frequently cited as a reason for hospital transfer, for example; some schedules urged the midwife to consider amniotomy where 'progress is slow'. Mandatory time limits were imposed on a woman during the second stage of her labour: 2 hours' pushing for a first baby, 1 hour for a second (Expert Group on Domiciliary Births, unpublished report, 1998).

HOME BIRTH LITIGATION

The 1970 Act obliged the State to provide free maternity care to all pregnant women, in hospital and outside it. In 1988, the Supreme Court reaffirmed women's entitlement to a home birth service, ruling that such services were to be provided under contract to the State. The applicant had sought a midwifery service, however:

---

[3] Domino scheme: a hospital midwifery scheme offering antenatal and intrapartum care (with early hospital discharge) and home postnatal care from the same team of midwives.

Mr Justice Finlay ruled that such services could – in law, if not in practice – be provided by general practitioners (*Spruyte and Wates* v. *Southern Health Board* [1988] JR 339). In the wake of the Dunne Case (*Dunne (infant)* v. *National Maternity Hospital* [1989] IR: 91; 1989 ILRM 735; cited in Tomkin & Hanafin 1995: 73), however, health boards began to discontinue their practice of contracting midwives to provide home birth services, offering grants to applicants instead. The 1980s and 1990s were marked by litigation, as parents – denied a grant by health boards – increasingly resorted to legal action to secure their rights. Some women, denied assistance by local boards, elected to have a professionally unattended home birth.

By 1999, aided by the public health system, obstetrics had its own, minuscule, home birth service. Health boards now began to invigilate midwifery practice in the community. Having discontinued the practice of entering into service agreements with midwives some years previously, the boards now argued that midwives were providing 'private' home birth services that were outside their control; before paying a grant, the boards told the courts, they would have to satisfy themselves that women were 'suitable' candidates for home birth. By mid-1999, such assessment had become a prerequisite for a grant in some areas.

Whether or not the boards were legally entitled to enforce eligibility criteria for home birth services was the nub of a High Court action in 1999 (*Nevin-Maguire and Maguire* v. *South-Eastern Health Board* [1999] JR 346). Marie Nevin-Maguire, a midwife, wished to have her sixth child at home, contrary to a local protocol: she had previously given birth to five children without difficulty; the Board refused her a service. An obstetrician testified that the Board's position ignored the fact that women having a sixth child do not face substantially increased risks of having an adverse outcome; rather, statistically, the risks increase slowly with successive births. The Board settled the case.

A raft of litigation followed on the same legal point, with home birth parents under the care of independent midwives refusing to be assessed for home birth by general practitioners, as demanded by bureaucrats. The latter seemed oblivious to the fact that general practitioners generally have 6 months' training, at most, in obstetrics and none in normal birth, an area of specialist practice in independent midwifery.

In the medical anxiety to control midwifery practice, distance from a mother's home to a consultant-controlled maternity unit (also cited in *Nevin-Maguire and Maguire* v. *South-Eastern Health Board*) became a major focus. In a case taken by four home birth mothers against three Dublin health boards (aborted prior to hearing), travel times of 20–70 minutes were cited as an 'unacceptable' risk in the High Court (*Bacon and others* v. *South-Western Area Health Board, South-Eastern Area Health Board and Northern Area Health Board* [2001] JR 665). In a previous, similar case rejected by the High Court (*Tarrade and others* v. *Northern Area Health Board* [2000] JR 184; [2003] IR 208), a medical practitioner alleged, wrongly, that home birth services could only be provided on behalf of the State by medical practitioners contracted to do so. None were willing, he said. Citing this allegation as fact, the Supreme Court denied the mothers' appeal ([2003] IR 208), ignoring its 1987 decision: the State, the judges ruled, was under no obligation to provide maternity care at home. The fact that midwives were equally empowered in law to provide home birth services on behalf of the State – and that some were more than willing to do so – was disregarded.

A 'STUDY' ON HOME BIRTH

Prior to the opening of the Supreme Court case, the 'findings' of a Rotunda Hospital 'study' on home birth in the eastern region (McKenna & Matthews 2003) were released as an 'exclusive' to a Sunday newspaper. 'Babies born at home 50 times more likely to die', screamed the banner headline (MacDonald 2003). A substantive critique (O'Connor et al 2003) found 'very poor quality data invalidating the authors' results'; it concluded that the Rotunda Hospital work was 'deeply skewed and quite misleading'.

Similarly, the noted British epidemiologist, Alison Macfarlane (2004) found 'no attempt to compare like with like: the authors' conclusions are therefore unfounded'. Figures bearing a remarkable resemblance to those published by McKenna & Matthews (2003) had first appeared in 2002, at an inquest into the death of a baby born at home.[4] These had been prepared at the coroner's request by another Rotunda consultant, a pathologist. Reintroduced in 2006, the figures (comparing death rates in home and hospital births) failed to convince: the jury returned a unanimous verdict that the infant had died of natural causes: they recommended 'more direct hospital contact, with full option of home birth still in place'.

COERCIVE STRATEGIES

Much has changed in the past decade. In the wake of the Kelly victory, a new determination to eliminate what William Arney ironically called the 'horror' of the medically unsupervised birth appeared. Regional groups (Condon 2000, for example) paid lip service to women's 'choice', even as they subverted it. These reports were premised on the self-serving medical view that midwifery practice is safe only under medical management.

This prejudicial view of midwifery found renewed favour in 2003, when the 1997 national group on domiciliary birth appeared in another guise, chaired by one of its former members, Sheila O'Malley. (As President of the Nursing Board, Ms O'Malley had unsuccessfully defended 17 High Court applications, three Supreme Court actions and a 4-year disciplinary hearing against Anne Kelly (see above).) The group devised a final solution to the problem of how to bring home birth mothers under medical management and independent midwives under

obstetric control (O'Malley, unpublished report, 2004). The new regulatory order promises to be one of the most draconian in the world: close supervision of midwives' clinical practice, including medical control of their client intake, is central to the proposed new regime. The O'Malley Report recommends that national, regional and local structures should 'determine access to hospital and laboratory services' (pp. 99–101): women's access to blood tests and ultrasound scans during pregnancy will be discretionary, hinging on 'access agreements between services and self-employed midwives', and grants, should they continue, 'should take cognizance of the presence of a second authorised practitioner' (O'Malley, unpublished report, 2004). Elsewhere, the O'Malley Report notes a clear need for 'ongoing' assessment 'during the confinement' (p. 92).

The view that a woman shall not be provided with midwifery services at home unless she is deemed medically suitable for such care represents a fundamental reversal of previous policy. In 1994, mindful of the fact that failure to provide a service had resulted in an 11% unattended home birth rate nationally (O'Connor 1995: 200), the McQuillan Group concluded: 'where a decision is made by a woman to give birth in her own home, health service personnel should respect that decision'.

An earlier draft of the O'Malley Report discusses the 'dilemma confronting health boards when a woman who does not satisfy the criteria . . . insists on having a home birth'. Two solutions are presented, the withdrawal of midwifery care during labour and forcible hospitalisation. The draft report notes that policy at the National Maternity Hospital is to seek a High Court order 'compelling the transfer of a patient to hospital' (O'Malley 2004: 12) 'for the safety of mother and unborn child'. The hospital is under the patronage of the Catholic Archbishop of Dublin.

A recent attempt by the hospital to coerce a prospective home birth mother into placing herself under its care failed, however. The mother had written to the Master with a birth plan for caesarean section, should she need one, if her physiological breech birth at home did not

---

[4] Note: this inquest (*Dublin County Coroner* [2006] *Re Baby Fogarty*) commenced in November 2002; adjourned because of a judicial review taken by a midwife challenging statistics introduced by the coroner, the inquest resumed (and concluded) on 10 January 2006.

succeed (P Canning, personal communication, 2006). She lived within 10 minutes' drive of the hospital. Following legal discussions between both sides, however, the Master abandoned his previously stated intention to seek a court order committing the woman to hospital prior to the onset of labour.

In another case in the west, the client of an independent midwife was forced to flee, at term, from her home during pregnancy, lest she be compelled to give birth in hospital. Michael Mylotte, the obstetric head of the hospital's domino/home birth scheme – himself a member of both the 1997 and 2003 home birth review groups – disagreed with the mother's decision to have a home birth, as she had an unstable lie and an ultrasound scan, according to Mylotte, showed a placenta praevia, a finding disputed by the ultrasonographer. Niamh Mulvaney subsequently gave birth without difficulty in rented accommodation some 130 miles from her home (N Mulvaney, personal communication, 2006).

Coercive measures have also been taken against home birth parents whose babies died in utero or after birth, and there have been several instances of enforced postmortems in Dublin. In one case, where a Potter's syndrome baby (whose congenital problems were incompatible with life) was born at home under the care of an independent midwife, a postmortem was carried out against the parents' express wishes by the National Maternity Hospital (N O Brolcháin, personal communication, 2006).

More recently, health authorities and hospitals have threatened parents wishing to exercise choice in healthcare, including place of birth, with child proceedings. One mother of three, living nearly 2 hours' drive from her nearest hospital, who had previously had a roadside birth, persisted in seeking a local maternity service from the State: she was threatened with a child protection order by a senior midwife at the National Maternity Hospital (L O'Shea, personal communication, 2005).

Coercive strategies, however, may be doomed to failure, as Irish courts frequently follow precedents set in other common law jurisdictions.

Courts in North America and England have decided that the law should not be used to coerce or restrict a pregnant woman in order to protect her fetus. While outside Ireland actions involving pregnant women have occasionally succeeded in the past, they are unlikely to do so in the future, if legal principles established in cases such as *St George's Healthcare NHS* v. *S* are upheld (Seymour 2000: 365).

RESTRICTING MIDWIFERY PRACTICE

More recently, obstetrics has found other ways to restrict midwifery practice in the community. In October 2002, Dublin obstetricians refused to scan a prospective home birth mother who developed bleeding at term: Consultants both at the National Maternity Hospital and the Coombe Women's Hospital declined to scan Laura Burrell unless she admitted herself as an inpatient; their hospitals, they told her, did not share care with self-employed midwives. Ms Burrell was a 'booked patient' at the National Maternity Hospital (L Burrell, personal communication, 2003).

In January 2003, citing 'vicarious liability' for patients, the National Maternity Hospital announced that it would no longer accept bloods for analysis from independent midwives, nor ultrasound referrals (D Keane, unpublished letter to the Home Birth Association, 2003). The other Dublin maternity hospitals eventually followed suit: all three are publicly funded, national specialist referral centres.

The claim that a hospital could be vicariously liable for an adverse event in a home birth attended by a self-employed midwife was subsequently rebutted. A senior legal advisor to the State Clinical Indemnity Scheme (K Rybaczuk, personal communication, 2004) judged the vicarious liability argument groundless. Nevertheless, the Dublin hospitals' ban on bloods and scans continues at the time of writing (A Murphy, personal communication, 2006). As in the Kelly case, professional power drives the issue. In a case aborted prior to hearing, Declan Keane testified that the difficulty is: 'lack of compliance by independent midwives with the Respondent's protocols' (*Home Birth Association of Ireland* v. *National Maternity Hospital and Eastern Regional Health Authority* [2003] JR 251).

Some family doctors have been advised not to accept prospective home birth mothers as patients. At least one insurer, Medisecc, has advised its general practitioner members not to accept such women for antenatal and postnatal care: yet their legal entitlement to free services (under the 1970 Act) depends on such acceptance.

The 1970 Health Act also obliges independent midwives to notify the local health authority annually in whose functional area they intend to practice. In June 2004, the Health Services Executive Western Area, while supportive of her clinical practice in the past, refused to accept a notification from an independent midwife. The authority declined to cite reasons for its refusal (C Engels, personal communication, 2005).

Over the past 10 years, the birth community in Ireland has succeeded in publicly establishing a counter discourse to obstetrics. Home birth, for example, is now rarely, if ever, discussed in the broadcast or print media from a solely medical perspective: debate has become the established norm. While childbirth groups have traditionally avoided politics, a new group, the National Birth Alliance, has been formed to campaign for women's rights in childbirth. With the 1985 Nurses' Act in the process of being rewritten and a new health act in the pipeline, lobbying is seen by some as the strategy of the future.

Finally, with medical bodies planning to close half of the country's maternity units (Comhairle na nOspidéal 2001: 29), it is difficult to believe that midwifery-based services, including home birth, will not ultimately form part of the core maternity services offered by the State to women.

RECLAIMING BIRTH

Legislative reform offers a way to resolve the conflicting views held by some women and the medical profession on birth, but achieving this goal will depend on the ability of women, and others who support a more natural approach to birth, to mobilise public opinion – and political support – for their views.

A FUTURE FOR HOME BIRTH?

Active management nearly succeeded in its goal to eliminate the midwifery model of birth. But as awareness of women's human rights in the birth chamber grows, midwives' consciousness of their rights as female professionals may expand. Secondly, both existing (Council Directive 86/613/EEC) and incoming equality directives from the European Union may strengthen their economic rights. Thirdly, women's right to refuse unwanted medical intervention may find a new pillar in the Human Rights Act 2004, enacting in Irish law the European Convention on Human Rights and Fundamental Freedoms.

CONCLUSION

As obstetrics strives to enforce its monopoly over the services for birth, using the language of risk to cloak a control agenda, risk has now become one of the dominant paradigms of our era, grist to the corporate mill of insurers and others.

In industrialised societies, women have lost the right to determine how – and where – to give birth (see Illich 1995 for an analogy: death under intensive care). The language of choice is used more and more to cloak its absence in an increasingly regulated environment. Obstetrics uses such rhetoric when it suits, to justify the performance of medically unnecessary caesarean sections, for example, but rarely champions women's decisions in the labour ward, where these conflict with obstetric policy.

Active management, a system that promoted a deeply prejudicial view of midwifery, enabled doctors to become monopoly providers in maternity care. The view that medically unsupervised midwifery practice is 'unsafe' has now taken root. Legal, regulatory and other barriers to midwifery practice restrict women's freedom in birth, while creating an environment for childbearing that is less than safe.

Today the boundaries between midwifery and medicine are set by multidisciplinary 'consensus' groups dominated by medical practitioners whose vested interests are rarely challenged. With the dominance of active management in hospital maternity care, home birth has become the last contested border between doctors and midwives, between normal and abnormal birth, between male medical speciali-sation and female midwifery expertise. Defining and policing the boundary around those few services still characterised by the midwifery model of care lies at the heart of the 'debate' between risk and choice.

Obstetrics employs the language of 'safety' to justify medical intervention when it is unwanted by women, while at the same time engaging in restrictive practices – withholding access to public hospital diagnostics to independent midwives, for example – that expose home birth mothers and their babies to greater risks during pregnancy. The continuing refusal of Dublin's three public maternity hospitals to supply blood tests and ultrasound scans to self-employed midwives' clients is a perversion of the public interest. The willingness of health authorities, public hospitals and medical consultants to jeopardise women's health in this way in the name of 'safety' suggests that power, not safety, is the driver. The use of coercive measures against home birth parents, such as the enforced postmortem carried out on a Potter's syndrome child born at home, reinforces the view that the place of birth debate is not about risk: it is about dominance.

Over the last decade, home birth policy has been driven by an overriding need to control the practice of independent midwives, employing the language of risk as a tool – copper-fastening obstetric revenues – to extend medical power into the home, at the cost of human rights to mothers and economic rights to midwives. Underlying the debate on the place of birth is a more fundamental question for society: who should control, and profit from, the services for maternity (O'Connor et al 2003).

Within a deeply patriarchal culture, medicine – unless checked – will continue to exercise an influence that is both inappropriate and disproportionate. Women who refuse to take medical advice are seen as challenging the authority of medicine and medical institutions. The safety and welfare of mother and baby are of primary importance, health authorities maintain, not a woman's right to decide how – and where – to give birth. Behaviour that is not medically sanctioned is invested with danger, real or imaginary: having a home birth contrary to medical advice is lambasted as irresponsible and selfish. But as the Dublin experience shows, medical technocrats – doctors and bureaucrats – take the view that self-regarding medical institutions must be protected, even at the expense of women's health during pregnancy, and that of their babies.

The repressive measures strategically devised by the O'Malley Group will, if implemented, erode an already minuscule home birth service, damaging even further an already haemorrhaging profession. Closing off the option of home birth in this way from 'unsuitable' women will inevitably result in a rise in professionally unattended births. Home birth will *not* be eradicated, as the 1993 survey found. As the McQuillan Report observed, it *is* unacceptable that any woman should feel compelled to give birth alone, without professional help. But today, it seems that the moral imperative to provide a health service to those in greatest need has evaporated.

Instead, a new willingness to coerce is evident, a belief that women can, and should, be compelled, if necessary, to accept medical treatment, however unwanted. However, as John Seymour underlines, child proceedings and fetal rights advocacy should have no part to play in ensuring health in childbirth. And, even if the ethics of coercion are to be ignored, the international legal climate has changed since the 1980s' vogue for forced caesareans. The past decade has seen the upholding, by both British and American courts, of a principle not fully understood or accepted (O'Connor 2001b) in maternity care: the right to bodily integrity.

Women's challenge to the medicalisation of childbirth is a challenge to the power of medicine in society to expropriate health. Enabling women to exercise their autonomy in childbirth should be the goal of midwives and doctors. But medical culture promotes the self-serving theology that only the medical view is the correct one.

Medicine, and particularly obstetrics, needs to recognise the legitimacy of other points of view. The future lies in partnership, not coercion. Midwifery is the only profession in childbirth that has partnership at its theoretical core (Guilliland & Pairman 1995). To allow that partnership to come into being, obstetrics needs to relinquish its monopoly over the services for birth.

There is no such thing as zero risk in birth, nor absolute knowledge. Mothers, like health professionals, make decisions based on risks that are relative. Women's right to determine how, as well as where, to give birth will ultimately, one hopes, be recognised as a human right, bringing society one step closer to dismantling the medical monopoly over birth and giving parity of esteem to the midwifery model of care.

Legal Cases

Bacon and others v. *South-Western Area Health Board, South-Eastern Area Health Board and Northern Area Health Board* [2001] JR 665

Dunne (infant) v. *National Maternity Hospital* [1989] IR 91; [1989] ILRM 735

Home Birth Association of Ireland v. *National Maternity Hospital and Eastern Regional Health Authority* [2003] JR 251

Nevin-Maguire and Maguire v. *South-Eastern Health Board* [1999] JR 346

Spruyte and Wates v. *Southern Health Board* [1988] JR 339

Re Baby Fogarty [2006] Inquest Dublin County Coroner's Court

Tarrade and others v. *Northern Area Health Board* [2000] JR 184; [2003] IR 208

References

Arney WR 1982 Power and the profession of obstetrics. Chicago University Press, Chicago

Bonham S 2005 Report on perinatal statistics for 2001. Economic and Social Research Institute, Dublin

Brenner H 2001 The National Maternity Hospital domino and hospital outreach home birth service pilot project evaluation. Women's Health Unit, Northern Area Health Board, Dublin, App 2

Brenner H 2004 Evaluation of the Southern Health Board home birth pilot project. In: O'Malley S. Domiciliary Births Group Report to the chief executive officers of the health boards (unpublished)

Cartwright E, Thomas J 2001 Constructing risk: maternity care, law and malpractice. In: De Vries R et al (eds) Birth by design: pregnancy, maternity care and midwifery in North America and Europe. Routledge, New York

Chamberlain G, Phillip E, Howlett B et al 1978 British births 1970: Vol 2 Obstetric care. Heinemann, London

Comhairle na nOspidéal (The Hospitals' Council) 1976 Development of hospital maternity services: a discussion document. Comhairle na nOspidéal, Dublin

Comhairle na nOspidéal 2001 Consultant staffing, January 2001. Comhairle na nOspidéal, Dublin

Commission on Nursing 1998 Report of the Commission on Nursing: a blueprint for the future. The Stationery Office, Dublin

Condon D 2000 Report of the Review Group on Maternity Services in the North-Eastern Health Board (unpublished)

Council Directive 86/613/EEC, 11 Dec 1986, on the application of the principle of equal treatment between men and women engaged in an activity, including agriculture, in a self-employed capacity and in the protection of self-employed women during pregnancy and motherhood. Online. Available: http://europa.eu.int/eur-lex/lex/LexUriServ/LexUriServ.do?uri=CELEX:31986L0613:EN:HTML

Cullen G 2002 Report on perinatal statistics for 1999. Economic and Social Research Institute, Dublin

Davis-Floyd RE 1992 Birth as an American rite of passage. University of California Press, Berkeley

Department of Health and Children 2000 North/South study of MRSA in Ireland 1999. Department of Health and Children, Dublin

Donnellan E 2004 The Irish Times, 15 Oct

European Workgroup of Independent Midwives 2000 Europe needs midwives: midwives and women for a healthier Europe. European Workgroup of Independent Midwives, Epen

Guilliland K, Pairman S 1995 The midwifery partnership: a model for practice. Monography Series: 95/1. Victoria University of Wellington, Wellington

Home Birth Association of Ireland Newsletter, Summer/Autumn 2005

Illich I 1995 Limits to medicine: medical nemesis, the expropriation of health, 2nd edn. Marian Boyers, London

Irish College of General Practitioners 1997 National general practice survey. Section 1: personal information. Irish College of General Practitioners, Dublin

Irish Independent 1992, 5 Apr

Kane E 1978 The last place God made: traditional economy and new industry in rural Ireland. Human Relations Area Files, Connecticut

Katz Rothman B 1982 In labour. Junction Books, London

MacDonald D 2003 Babies born at home 50 times more likely to die. Sunday Times, 31 Aug

Macfarlane A 2004 Safety of home and hospital birth – data does (sic) not support the conclusions. Letter. Irish Medical Journal 2004: 96(4). Online. Available: www.imj.ie

McKenna P, Matthews T 2003 Safety of home delivery compared with hospital delivery in the Eastern Regional Health Authority in Ireland in the year 1999–2002. Irish Medical Journal 2003: 96(7). Online. Available: www.imj.ie

McQuillan P 1994 Report of the Maternity and Infant Care Scheme Review Group. Department of Health, Dublin

Murphy-Lawless J 1989 Male texts and female bodies: the colonisation of childbirth by men midwives. In: Torode B (ed) Text and talk as social practice. Foris, Amsterdam

Murphy-Lawless J 1998 Reading birth and death: a history of obstetric thinking. Cork University Press, Cork

Obstetric Working Group, National Health Insurance Board of the Netherlands 2000 Obstetric manual: final report of the Obstetric Working Group of the National Health Insurance Board of the Netherlands. Online. Available: www.cvz.np/Downloads/Publicaties/verB-vad.pdf.

O'Connell R, Cronin M 2002 Home birth in Ireland 1993–1997: a review of community midwifery practice. All-Ireland Journal of Nursing and Midwifery, Apr

O'Connor M 1995 Birth tides: turning towards home birth. Pandora, London

O'Connor M 2001a Equal rights in the birth chamber: the need for a midwife-based system of maternity care in Europe. MIDIRS Midwifery Digest Mar 11(1): 129–132

O'Connor M 2001b Forced labour: how we manage women in childbirth. The Irish Times, 13 Aug. Online. Available: www.ireland.com (subscribers only)

O'Connor M, Canning P, Rybaczuk K 2003 Safety of home delivery compared with hospital delivery in the Eastern Regional Health Authority in Ireland in the year 1999–2002. Abstract writers' comments. MIDIRS Midwifery Digest 13(4): 515–518

O'Driscoll K, Meagher D, Boylan P 1993 Active management of labor, 3rd edn. Mosby, London

O'Malley S 2004 Domiciliary Births Group Report to the chief executive officers of the health boards, Dec (unpublished)

Park L 2005 Who's regulating whom? Midwifery Matters, Summer: 9–12

Pfeufer Kahn R 1995 Bearing meaning: the language of birth. University of Illinois Press, Urbana

Porter R 2000 Home is where the heart is . . . and the head? Home Birth Association of Ireland Conference, Dublin, Ireland, Apr

Seymour J 2000 Childbirth and the law. Oxford University Press, Oxford

The Nurses' Act 1985. The Stationery Office, Dublin

Tomkin D, Hanafin P 1995 Irish medical law. Round Hall Press, Dublin

Wertz R, Wertz D 1977 Lying-In: a history of childbirth in America. Free Press, New York

Wiley MM, Merriman B 1997 Women & health care in Ireland. Oak Tree Press/ESRI, Dublin

Williams AS 1997 Women and childbirth in the twentieth century. Sutton, Stroud

Witz A 1992 Professions and patriarchy. Routledge, London

Endnote

Based on 61684 births in 2004, ex 23913 in Dublin (www.cso.ie/statistics/bthsdthsmarriages.htm); a public/private/semi-private ratio of 50:25:25; and 45 obstetricians in Dublin, where private fees average an estimated €3000, dropping to €2000 elsewhere and a fixed semi-private fee of €790.

Chapter **11**

Risk Perception and Analysis in Australia

Jennifer Cameron and David Ellwood

INTRODUCTION

The notions of risk and choice are closely inter-twined because the way in which risk is perceived and analysed will influence the perception of, and the availability of, choices. In Slovic's view, whoever controls the definition of risk controls the solutions to be acted on the perceived risk (Slovic 1999). In Australia there are several points of input in the governance of maternity services. The stakeholders involved include the various government departments such as health and community services and the professional registration/regulatory bodies; the professional/standard setting bodies; the clinicians, medical and midwifery; managers and teachers; and the consumers.

Chapters 11 and 12 will explore risk and choice from the Australian perspective. In Chapter 11 factors influencing the perception and analysis of risk will be examined, and in Chapter 12 how choices are enacted, incorporating the processes of collaboration and the use of reflection, will be explored.

THE AUSTRALIAN SETTING

DEMOGRAPHIC DETAILS

Australia covers 7.7 million km². It is the driest continent on earth with around one-third considered desert. It is approximately 3700 km long (north to south) and 4000 km wide.

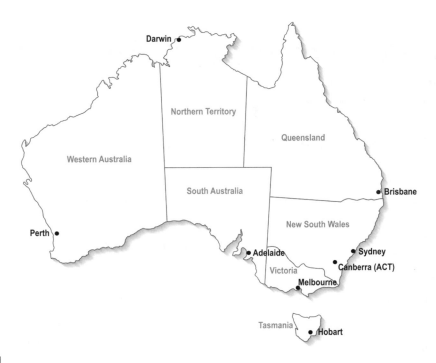

Figure 11.1

The mainland comprises five states and two territories. The sixth state, Tasmania, is 200 km south of Victoria and separated from the mainland by Bass Strait. Australia is the largest island, the smallest continent and the only nation to occupy an entire continent. The mainland section is roughly divided in the east by the Great Dividing Range which lies inland from the eastern seaboard and runs from the Cape York Peninsula in Queensland to Melbourne in Victoria. Included in the range is Australia's highest peak, Mount Kosciusko (2229 m) near the New South Wales (NSW)-Victoria border in the snow-capped alpine region of the Great Dividing Range. West of the dividing range the land is mainly flat with a few low ranges including the Flinders Ranges in South Australia and the MacDonnell Ranges near Alice Springs. The centre of the continent is mainly desert and sparsely populated.

Around 80% of the Australian population lives within the eastern seaboard or the coastal fringes of the continent. Australia is a multicultural society with a dominant Western lifestyle. Only 2.4% of Australia's population identifies as Aboriginal and/or Torres Strait Islander, our indigenous people. Approximately 65% of indigenous Australians live in towns and cities with the remainder occupying rural and remote areas.

The Northern Territory (NT) has the largest proportion of its population who are indigenous; approximately 29% (see Table 1). Indigenous people are more likely to live in remote areas than the non-indigenous population. This creates significant access and equity healthcare issues which affect choice for indigenous women and their families and communities.

BIRTH STATISTICS

Approximately 250 000 babies are born in Australia each year. The following figures represent statistics for the year 2002:

Of babies born in 2002, 2.3% were born with the aid of assisted reproductive technology (ART). Almost half of these babies were born by caesarean section (49.4%), had a lower average

Table 11.1   Population breakdown by state/territory and indigenous status

Total population State/Territory	Number (thousands)		Proportion of state & territory population (%)	Proportion of total indigenous population (%)
		Indigenous population		
New South Wales	6575.2	134.9	2.1	29.4
Victoria	4804.7	27.8	0.6	6.1
Queensland	3628.9	125.9	3.5	27.5
South Australia	1511.7	25.5	1.7	5.6
Western Australia	1901.2	65.9	3.5	14.4
Tasmania	471.8	17.4	3.7	3.8
Northern Territory	197.8	56.9	28.8	12.4
Australian Capital Territory	319.3	3.9	1.2	0.9
Australia	19413.2	458.5	2.4	100.0

Australian Bureau of Statistics Census 2001

Total number of births	255 095
Births by caesarean section	27.6%
Average age at first birth	27.9
Indigenous mothers	8822 (3.6%)
Indigenous mothers in the NT	38.4%
Perinatal mortality rate	9.8:1000
Maternal mortality rate	10:100 000

For indigenous people the rates are worse (from Laws & Sullivan 2004).

Perinatal mortality rate	21.8:1000
Maternal mortality rate	34.8:100 000

birth weight compared with the average Australian baby and 20.9% were born preterm. At least some of these increases in intervention and adverse outcomes can be explained by the higher rate of multiple pregnancies. As the average age of childbirth continues to rise (Laws & Sullivan 2004), it seems inevitable that this trend will continue, presenting maternity and perinatal services with particular increased risks and challenges.

HISTORICAL PERSPECTIVES

Currently Australia has a two-tiered healthcare system. A national health insurance system, Medicare, is funded by the Commonwealth government through a compulsory tax levy.

Medicare provides free public hospital care, an 85% rebate of the schedule (recommended) fee for in-hospital care for private patients, and also reimburses 75% of out of hospital medical and some allied healthcare costs. Private health insurance is available and is purchased by approximately 40% of Australians (Private Health Insurance Administration Council 2005). Private health insurance allows choice of specialist and covers hospital costs in both private and public hospitals. There are now significant tax incentives and penalties designed to encourage women to take out private health insurance, as well as a 'safety net' which covers out of pocket medical expenses once these have risen above $1000 per annum ($500 if in a low income bracket). These recent changes can, in part, explain the gradual shift towards private maternity care which can now be considered to be heavily subsidised by the Commonwealth. Changes to the fee structures of obstetricians has meant the women can claim back a large proportion of the costs incurred for private maternity care. This has had a number of impacts on maternity services. There is no longer any control on fees exerted by market forces so these can rise disproportionately. Secondly, the shift to private maternity care is continuing to drive the rates of certain interventions such as induction of labour and caesarean section. Interestingly, apart from a small number of health funds, there are no rebates for midwifery-based maternity services. Consequently, at a time when private obstetric care is flourishing under current government policy, independent midwifery practice is struggling to survive due to the lack of availability of indemnity insurance and the fact that all costs are carried by the woman choosing this model of care.

History of Maternity Services in Australia

In Australia the States and Territories have managed their own health services with financial input from the Commonwealth and as a result maternity services differ between the States and Territories. Willis (1989) presents an in-depth history of increasing medical dominance over the area of childbirth continuing until very recently. Tensions also existed between nursing and midwifery which resulted in the subordination of midwifery by nursing. Nurses' boards were dominated by medical interests and the scope of practice of midwives became restricted along with women's choice of caregiver.

By the 1920s, the above changes plus alterations to funding arrangements meant that all women had to seek private health insurance to be admitted to a hospital; only the very poor could obtain a limited free service in public hospitals, the only place where they could access maternity care. As well, only doctors had visiting rights to hospitals, thus women were locked into hospital birth under medical care (Reiger 2003).

In the late 1960s and early 1970s the Childbirth Education Association developed a strong consumer voice and lobbied for reform in maternity services. A gradual groundswell of support followed, culminating in several states commissioning reviews of their birthing and/or obstetric services. Several publications followed (DoH NSW 1989, Health Department Victoria 1990, NT DoH 1992,) Western Australia (WA), Legislative Assembly Select Committee 1995). Various federal government reviews were commissioned, *Options for Effective Care in Childbirth* in 1996; *Review of the Services Offered by Midwives* in 1998 (both National Health and Medical Research Council) and *Rocking the Cradle: A Senate Report into Childbirth Procedures* in 1999 (Senate Community Affairs Reference Committee).

In spite of the results of all these reviews demonstrating the need for, and the safety of, alternative models of maternity care, little was implemented. Public support continued and in 2002 the National Maternity Action Plan was prepared and released by several community organisations. This plan was presented to State, Territory and Federal governments as the blueprint for future maternity services for Australia. Finally, the recommendations of all these reviews are only just beginning to be implemented and are at various stages in the states and territories. At the time of writing this chapter Victoria (July 2004) and the Northern Territory (November 2004) had announced plans to reform maternity services with the option of the midwife as the primary carer for well women, and continuation of options for care from a general practitioner (GP) or private obstetrician.

CURRENT MODELS OF CARE AND STRUCTURE

Australian maternity services may be located in major metropolitan hospitals, outer metropolitan and regional hospitals, rural and remote areas and less than 1% of births take place at home (Laws & Sullivan 2004). A search using the internet will reveal the many models of care available currently in Australia. Broadly these

Table 11.2   Place of birth, all confinements, by state and territory, 2002

Place of birth	NSW	Vic	Qld	WA	SA	Tas	ACT	NT	Aus
Hospital	82 149	80 185	47 617	23 913	16 318	5528	4427	3593	243 730
Birth centre	2024	1429	389	278	1000	6	253	–	5379
Home	99	163	61	121	47	n.p	14	17	522
Other	315	246	257	84	56	76	14	54	1112
Not stated	–	–	–	–	–	15	–	–	15
Total	84 587	62 023	48 324	24 396	17 421	5625	4708	3674	250 758

Laws & Sullivan 2004

can be categorised as primary, secondary and tertiary level services in the public health system and private maternity services. Primary level services are slowly being implemented in most states and territories of Australia. Most care takes place within the secondary and tertiary levels with public hospital care being the most common, offering several care modalities. These include team midwifery, consultant care, shared care (community GP and midwife/obstetrician), a mixed care model (resident doctors/-midwives/consultants) and community case-load midwifery. Births may take place in the standard public hospital setting or birth centre or at home.

Privately insured women may receive care from an obstetrician, GP, a midwife or a combination thereof. The place of birth is usually in a hospital setting with the few births that occur at home being most likely attended by a midwife. The rising cost of professional indemnity insurance has forced most general practitioners and privately practising midwives out of the market, thus reducing choices for women, particularly home birth with a midwife. This is in spite of good outcomes from birth at home or in a birth centre with midwife-led care.

Outcomes and Model of Care

A recent large study conducted in NSW revealed that rates of obstetric intervention for privately insured women birthing in private hospitals far exceeded those of women receiving publicly funded care and exceeded those of privately

insured women birthing in a public hospital (Roberts et al 2000). Both groups studied were at low risk of complications. The most significant finding was that privately insured women birthing in private hospitals had high rates of instrumental births; they also had higher rates of epidural analgesia, induction and augmentation. This may mean that privately insured women birthing in private hospitals have more available choice such as epidural on demand. The irony is that the most affluent women have the highest interventions and are at higher risk of adverse outcomes such as those associated with instrumental birth.

Community Midwifery Programmes

Currently there are several community midwifery programmes running in Australia. In WA the community midwifery practice has been in operation for 9 years, having commenced in 1996 (http://www.communitymidwives.org.au/cmp/history.htm). Outcomes are excellent and the service is in demand. The WA model has been used as a template for future models in other states and territories. Thus risk and choice in childbirth in Australia are greatly influenced by the model of maternity care.

RISK MANAGEMENT IN AUSTRALIA

Modern health service risk management began in earnest in Australia with the NSW and Victorian Law Reform Commissions' publications *Informed Decisions about Medical Procedures*. In 1989 The Australian National Health and

Medical Research Council were asked to formulate guidelines about proposed treatments and procedures and in 1993 *General Guidelines for Medical Practitioners on providing Information to Patients* was published. In 2000, in response to global trends, the Australian Council for Safety and Quality in Health Care was established and state and territory governments set up Clinical Risk Management Committees.

With specific reference to maternity services, most of the work on standards, and collection of clinical indicators has been done outside of direct government influence. The Australian Council on Healthcare Standards (ACHS) developed a range of clinical indicators in conjunction with the Royal Australian College of Obstetricians and Gynaecologists in 1992. Shortly after this a group called Women's Hospitals of Australasia (WHA) was founded to provide, amongst other activities, a forum for benchmarking between similar hospitals. Membership of WHA is voluntary and costs member hospitals an annual fee to take part. Nevertheless, more than 30 of the larger maternity units in Australia and New Zealand have been members and contributed to two *Benchmarking in Obstetrics* publications in recent times (Buist & Cahill 2004). These have covered a wide range of clinical indicators including some uncommon, but serious adverse outcomes such as peripartum hysterectomy. More recently, WHA's activities have been extended to include the development of national care guidelines, the running of annual clinical forums to deal with 'hot topics' such as smoking in pregnancy and postpartum haemorrhage

Despite there being considerable activity within these bodies and others such as Royal Australian and New Zealand College of Obstetricians and Gynaecologists (RANZCOG), and Australian College of Midwives Incorporated (ACMI), there is no national, government-sponsored body which is primarily concerned with standards of maternity care, or accreditation of maternity units. Linking this kind of activity with the collection of national perinatal statistics (currently done by the Australian Institute of Health & Welfare through its National Perinatal Statistics Unit) would seem to be a

logical next step. Ideally, this should involve the colleges involved in the various professional disciplines who deliver maternity care. A national guidelines unit would also help to remedy the current situation where there are many different bodies involved in guideline development and propagation.

FACTORS INFLUENCING PERCEPTION OF RISK IN AUSTRALIAN MATERNITY SERVICES

Risk is generally defined as 'the potential for unwanted outcome' (Wilson 1994). All pregnancies face risk and risk during childbearing is defined as the probability of (the mother or the baby) dying or experiencing serious injury as a result of the pregnancy (WHO 1998). Even with the best risk-screening tools it is impossible to accurately predict who will need what level of service. Therefore it is important that all women have access to high quality essential maternity services.

Risk is perceived differently by practitioners and consumers. In two UK studies (McGeary 1994, Heaman et al 1992) there was no relationship between self-rated pregnancy risk and the biomedical risk score. In one study (McGeary 1994), women who were designated as high risk according to a medical risk score did not perceive themselves to be at high risk. Perception will also be influenced by the person's belief or perception of their health status.

A recent study in Australia, the Australian Patient Safety Survey, demonstrated that several factors influenced patients' perception of risk (Clarke 2004: 50–51). Higher education and a higher income resulted in a feeling of being safe and thus comfortable to 'take a risk', as did having a regular doctor. Those who reported being informed of the benefits and limitations of a treatment were more likely to view hospitals as safe settings; this was independent of education or income. Females were more likely than males to view hospitals as places of potential risk, particularly the age group 25–54. Perceptions about the risks or pain associated with childbirth were thought to be associated factors. Perhaps pain or the possibility of having procedures inflicted on a perceived 'healthy' body is seen as more risky than if the body was 'ill' or 'unhealthy', although this does not explain the high rates of intervention amongst privately insured women.

In the same study it was found that most females preferred a participative, informed model of decision-making in healthcare. Bastian (2003) explains that although the Australian community in general is healthier than ever, people appear to be afraid of risks; almost as if risk is equated with problem. The way risk is communicated will greatly influence the way a woman perceives her risk factor.

COMMUNICATING RISK

Risk communication is essential and the way risk is perceived will be influenced by the person's perception of health and this in turn will be influenced by factors such as race and culture. As Bastian (2003) states, there is no 'one size fits all' guideline in communicating risk to women/patients and assisting women to make a balanced choice. In Australia, indigenous people balance their risks within a framework of cultural and community needs and values. There is no such concept as percentage in indigenous language and so the use of percentages is meaningless in trying to convey the concept of risk (Trudgen 2000). This is important to be aware of when explaining health information to indigenous Australians. While it is now becoming more accepted that standard (medical) ways of explaining risk may not be appropriate to indigenous women, the same also applies to many other groups within the Australian community. Recently, there has been some success demonstrated with the use of decision-aids for explaining choices, particularly when this involves balancing risks. This has been demonstrated recently with a randomised trial of a decision-aid for women considering their options when faced with a breech presentation in the late third trimester (Nassar et al in press). There are plans to extend this kind of methodology to other situations such as choosing elective caesarean section. However,

one of the real challenges is to develop methods of communicating risk (and choices) to women who are faced with rapid decision-making in an acute setting.

INFLUENCE OF GOVERNMENTS AND GOVERNANCE BODIES

Federal, state and territory governments and regulatory bodies influence risk and choice for Australian families. In 2002 in response to worldwide events and the possible collapse of the nation's biggest insurer, United Medical Protection, obstetricians found themselves facing the future without a satisfactory form of professional indemnity insurance. The federal government was quick to step in and provide $600 million to underwrite insurance for the obstetricians to enable them to maintain their private practices. No such assistance was provided for the midwives who practised privately.

In 2001 the providers of indemnity insurance to Australian midwives withdrew their cover. This resulted in privately practising midwives with no option but to practise uninsured or cease to practise privately. A further blow was struck when some of the Nursing and Midwifery Boards instigated mandatory professional indemnity insurance as a requirement for registration or renewal of registration for nurses and midwives. As there is currently no professional indemnity insurance available in Australia for midwives to purchase, this resulted in the inability to practise privately in the community for midwives. Midwives practising in institutions are partly covered by the institution and through membership of the Australian Nurses Federation (ANF). ANF purchases an insurance package to cover all members but the insurers will only cover midwives who practise in institutions, whether public or private, but not midwives who maintain private community practices. This means privately practising midwives are unable to run childbirth education classes in the community but other allied health professionals such as physiotherapists or dieticians may do so. For indigenous women in particular this had major ramifications for their cultural safety. As stated by a retired Senior Indigenous Health Worker in the Northern Territory:

> *You listen to us. It's very important for young girls to be able to have their babies in their communities if they want to, with their families and the midwife there together. It's up to them. Young mothers need to have their aunties and grandmothers with them to tell them what to do – our culture way.*
>
> (Wardaguga 2004)

In the Northern Territory this situation was ameliorated by its government agreeing to indemnify the privately practising midwives by employing them in a community midwifery model. Midwives who wish to practise independently of government-funded agencies do not have access to this cover, thus limiting choice for women and employment for the midwives.

LEGAL INFLUENCES

In Australia standards of informed consent are underpinned by the 1992 legal case 'Rogers v. Whitaker' (McPhee 2002). In *Rogers* v. *Whitaker* the court determined that an ophthalmic surgeon should have warned his patient of the 1:14 000 chance of going blind in the opposite eye due to the proposed procedure. This decision has profoundly influenced medical and health practice. Ultimately it is the decision of the patient whether or not to undergo a procedure and in order to make an informed choice the risks and benefits of the procedure, the risks and benefits of not having the procedure and the risks and benefits of any other options must be provided by the health practitioner. Meeting this obligation entails a thorough and clear explanation in a language the patient understands.

This puts a heavy onus on the midwife or doctor to cover all the requirements of informed consent and ensure that it is understood by the woman. The better a practitioner knows the woman, the more likely it is that the language will be acceptable and understood by her. Current models of care do not provide time for lengthy explanations. In response, some state governments have set up websites with evidence-based information presented for public use. In Victoria a web page has been set up by the Department of Human Services to provide Victorian families with information regarding their pregnancy and birth care (http://www.health.vic.gov.au/maternity/index.htm). The information provided is based on the best available evidence and is updated regularly. Terms like 'low risk' and 'high risk' are explained along with other research language.

MEDIA INFLUENCES

Media reports are often one-sided and ill informed, as well as driven by personal agendas. A recent media report in response to the announcement of plans to reorganise Victoria's maternity services and increase midwife-led births claimed that women would be dying by the roadside as a result (Kelly 2004). The reporter interviewed an obstetrician but failed to acknowledge that midwives were the most appropriate carers for healthy pregnant women. With a midwife in attendance, women would not have to travel long distances to give birth. As Swan (2005) has argued, some of the major Australian media outlets fall short of the standards required to support decision-making in the community.

In recent times there have been a number of major inquiries set up in relation to clinical services provided by hospitals, and the media has usually had a significant role in driving both community and political opinion about the problems. The recent Douglas Inquiry into maternity services in Western Australia's major teaching hospital (King Edward Memorial Hospital) came about, in part, due to the highly emotive publicity given to a number of cases with adverse outcomes reported by the local press. While the report did highlight many deficiencies in the risk management practices at that hospital, the impact of the media reporting on the morale of the clinical staff may well have had a significant negative effect on the way in which services were being delivered.

By evoking 'knee-jerk' responses by politicians looking for quick fixes to perceived problems, the media can frequently be seen to restrict choices to women, particularly if community concerns are raised about levels of risk which may not be real. This problem has been highly evident in Australia in recent times, particularly in relation to midwifery-led units, homebirth and other examples of low-intervention birthing.

STAKEHOLDER NOTIONS OF RISK

Indigenous Australians

Indigenous Australians perceive risk within their own language and culture. Indigenous people who may speak English conceptualise and think in their own language (Trudgen 2000). This has major implications for risk and choice during childbearing. For indigenous Australians health encompasses the social, emotional, spiritual and cultural wellbeing of an individual together with community capacity and governance and it is spiritually and culturally important to birth 'on country' (National ATSI Health Council 2001) (this means giving birth on the land the woman was born on and with other known women by her side). Indigenous women feel that their relationship to the land, established through the birthing experience, is vitally important to their culture and risk is perceived within this framework where to birth elsewhere, such as in a Western hospital, can lead to feeling culturally unsafe (Kildea et al 2004). For some indigenous women there is a special ceremony associated with the disposal of the placenta and membranes and if this ceremony is not carried out appropriately mothers and babies are weakened:

> It would make the mothers and babies healthier and stronger if we did the smoking ceremony. They should do that (Mary, Nancy and Marie).
>
> (Kildea et al 2004)

At present, in the top end of the Northern Territory, large amounts of money are spent transferring well indigenous women to Darwin (the capital city) to birth, on the grounds that it is safer than birthing in a remote or rural community; not only is this a misuse of public health money but it may result in serious cultural and emotional morbidity for these women and their communities. For the health managers, risk is perceived as the possibility of an unforeseen emergency and must be avoided at all cost; but for indigenous women risk is balanced against important cultural values and traditions. Kildea et al (2004) state that some indigenous women feel that giving birth in hospital is a cause of infant mortality. As a result of not being welcomed properly into the world by the appropriate ceremonies, the baby's weakened spirit gets sick. According to the indigenous women: 'The culture is still very important; following the rules keeps us strong, if you don't, then you get sick' (Kildea et al 2004).

The consequences are as illustrated:

> Some Indigenous women are performing their own 'risk assessment' and decide against leaving their homes and families for birth, preferring to present to the local health centre in strong labour, when it is too late to be transferred.
>
> (Kildea et al 2004)

In essence, the service provider's perspective incorporates concerns about the physical effects that potential problems will have on the service. Concerns include the risk of: something going wrong; delays in transport; litigation; rising professional indemnity costs; difficulty in maintaining skilled staffing around the clock (Kildea 2001). Indigenous women make their decisions within a social and cultural community setting, meeting not only their needs but also their family and community.

GENERAL NOTIONS OF RISK AMONG AUSTRALIAN WOMEN

Australia is a very multicultural society and it is difficult to define a risk framework to reflect the general public women's view. In recent years there has been a strong consumer voice advocating for change in Australian birthing services, bringing women back into the centre of birthing. The results of many reviews are beginning to be implemented and some women are able to lead their care in pregnancy and childbirth. For some women this will mean choosing a techno-medical birth where they can plan and control. For others it will mean being able to choose birth in the safety of their own home with a known and trusted caregiver.

MIDWIVES' NOTIONS OF RISK

The midwifery philosophy views birth as a normal life event. The ACMI (2005) states midwifery is founded on respect for women and on a strong belief in the value of women's work of bearing and rearing each generation. Midwifery considers women in pregnancy, during childbirth and early parenting to be undertaking healthy processes that are profound and precious events in each woman's life. The midwife works in partnership with the woman. The Australian College of Midwives governs professional midwifery in Australia and has clear guidelines for consultation and referral (ACMI 2003). One privately practising midwife in Australia proceeds as follows:

At the complementary 'getting to know you' visit I usually ask that the couple have any questions they may like to ask of me written down so we are less likely to forget any issues. Usually the sheet of questions with answers provided is filed in the couple's pregnancy record folder if they decide to contract with me to attend their home birth. I take along the home birth statistics for Australia, the perinatal statistics that compare outcomes in the various health areas in our state and a copy of Marjorie Tew's book 'Safer Childbirth?' and we have a general talk on evidence-based practice. I usually leave a list of websites where the couple can obtain further information so they can start to do more research for themselves as the pregnancy advances.

Inside the woman's pregnancy record folder is 'The Pregnant Woman's Bill of Rights and Responsibilities', a blank Birth Plan especially structured for my home birth clients and a 'Statement of Practice' that explains how my independent practice operates. As we continue with the prenatal visits more data is entered

into the couple's birth plan and potential risks of each stage of the pregnancy, birth or aftermath are elaborated on. I also have a client evaluation form that is completed AFTER I have finished seeing the couple.

(Robinson 2005, personal communication)

Ideally the midwife aims to follow each woman across the interface between institutions and the community, through pregnancy, labour and birth and the postnatal period so all women remain connected to their social support systems; the focus is on the woman, not on the institutions or the professionals involved (ACMI 2005). This is the framework within which most Australian midwives conceptualise risk. As noted by Reiger (2000), although contemporary [Australian] midwifery uses the discourse of women's 'choice' in different ways, the central tenet of woman-centred care prevails. Midwives acknowledge that some women will request a highly technical birth and informed consent is the key factor (Reiger 2000).

MEDICAL PRACTITIONERS' NOTIONS OF RISK

The RANZCOG has a role in setting the standards for obstetric practice in Australia. The RANZCOG mission statement is to pursue excellence in the delivery of healthcare to women throughout their lives. The principal ways in which it maintains standards of obstetric practice is through training of junior doctors in the practice of obstetrics and gynaecology, and by running continuing professional development programmes (CPD) for qualified specialists. Both the training and CPD programmes have been held up as excellent examples of professional adult learning during accreditation by the Australian Medical Council. Nevertheless, there remain significant tensions between obstetricians and other health professionals involved in maternity care.

There have been a number of attempts over recent times to work collaboratively with GPs (who provide many of the maternity services in rural Australia) and midwives, notably through the Joint Consultative Committee on Maternity Services. However, this positive approach to working together has often stalled when trying to share a common understanding of risk and choice in relation to birthing.

It is likely that most medical practitioners develop their own sense of risk and choice during their years as medical students and whilst training as junior doctors. One recent significant development in Australia has been the introduction of a Women's Health Core Curriculum, written by a consortium of clinical academics from many of the country's medical schools. This effort has now resulted in a standard textbook on Women's Health which has been endorsed by RANZCOG and is likely to become the standard text for Australian medical students. Perhaps this approach may provide an opportunity for introducing to medical students the concept that risk and choice are viewed from many different perspectives in relation to childbirth.

RISK ANALYSIS

Risk analysis generally takes place within the framework of acute care. Most births in Australia take place in an acute care facility and even if the woman starts with a community GP the process he/she follows will be set by the local hospital. In general, healthcare professionals use statistical data to determine the degree of risk and pregnant women use their own personal data, based on past and present conditions (Heaman et al 2004).

In Australia there are various tools for professional risk analysis. Most healthcare institutions use the principles of clinical risk management; peer review; analysis of incident data and root cause analysis in order to monitor and determine risk and set standards. Guidelines are reviewed regularly and are based on evidence for best practice.

Performance indicators are set by state governments and usually reflect the standards set by the ACHS. The indicators are used to measure the outcomes of maternity care. When analysing risk, these indicators will form the framework for the risk assessment process. Current indicators include rates of induction of labour; vaginal delivery following previous caesarean section, low Apgar scores, intact perineum rates and others. As discussed above, there is a move through the WHA to develop indicators of severe adverse outcome such as intensive care unit (ICU) admission, peripartum hysterectomy and severe postpartum haemorrhage.

THE INFLUENCE OF RESEARCH ON RISK ANALYSIS

Research findings have influenced maternity care in Australia. In 2000 the results of the term breech trial were published (Hannah et al 2000). The major finding was that planned caesarean section conferred better immediate perinatal outcomes for the baby. As a result, women with a breech-presenting infant were recommended caesarean section as the mode of birth, regardless of parity and previous births. The methodological flaws of this study have since been elucidated but only after many women have undergone caesarean section (Kotaska 2004). The RANZCOG has acknowledged this issue in a recent college statement (2005). RANZCOG states that while planned caesarean section is the safest mode of birth for most breech-presenting infants, there exists a small sub-group of women who will do extremely well with vaginal breech birth. In particular, those who wish to have a large family may be better advised to choose vaginal birth as having a scar in the uterus increases the risk of placenta praevia, and placenta accreta with its inherent increased risk of serious morbidity and mortality.

Research such as the term breech trial may have resulted in women viewing caesarean section as a procedure without risk. More Australian women are choosing caesarean section as their preferred mode of birth (Molloy 2004). Various explanations exist for this choice: many are for social reasons such as the need for a planned birth, others are for perceived improved pelvic floor integrity. The latter is not supported by research evidence. It is difficult to argue with a woman who has chosen to birth by caesarean section although there is an overwhelming professional and ethical responsibility to ensure that she is making an informed choice. If the notion of choice is to be supported as long as she is provided with the benefits and harms of the procedure it can be argued that it is her right to choose. For some practitioners fear of litigation will prevail: if I refuse on grounds there is no medical indication for the procedure and the baby is harmed I will be sued, therefore I will perform the caesarean section.

There are a number of randomised trials currently being conducted in Australia and New Zealand, involving a network of tertiary centres, coordinated through the Perinatal Clinical Trials Unit in Adelaide. Many of these may further influence perceptions of risk and choice once the results are available. These include a trial comparing vaginal birth after caesarean (VBAC) with planned elective caesarean section, and a study on the timing of birth in twins which involves a comparison of elective delivery at 37 weeks. There has been some resistance to both of these trials, particularly the first concerning VBAC, as it is thought that the results may be used in the same way as the term breech trial, to further restrict birthing choices for women. There remains this ethical paradox, whereby the responsibility to generate evidence from clinical trials to properly inform women, has to be balanced with the desire to maintain choices for women. Regardless of the evidence, some women will still choose a particular method of giving birth, accepting a small increased risk. If the impact of the trial is to close off this choice completely (as has happened with vaginal breech), rather than to provide evidence for women to consider when making their own choice, then the desirability of this outcome needs to be considered up-front. This has been argued strongly in relation to a 'Term Cephalic' trial of primary elective caesarean section versus vaginal birth (Robson & Ellwood 2003).

REACTIVE AND PROACTIVE RISK MANAGEMENT

It has been argued that there has been a gradual move away from reactive risk management in relation to childbirth, to proactive risk management. From the trainee's perspective, this means anticipating risk and avoiding the adverse outcome rather than being trained to deal with it, should it occur. This change in philosophy has both positive and negative results. On the positive side, it is clearly better to avoid the risk completely rather than have to deal with the problem. An example of this could be given concerning shoulder dystocia. A junior trainee over 20 years ago would have been taught how to deal with shoulder dystocia if it arose (reactive management). This is still the case today, although both obstetrics and gynaecology trainees and midwives are being trained in a more comprehensive way through courses such as Advanced Life Support in Obstetrics (ALSO). However, increasingly women with larger babies are being delivered by elective caesarean section to avoid this relatively uncommon event (proactive management). The negative side of this is that many caesarean sections need to be done to avoid one case of shoulder dystocia. Another negative impact is that the unexpected event becomes so uncommon that practitioners have lost the skills to deal with it. This may well have become the case for vaginal breech births, as recent graduates now have little experience of this method of delivery so are not as well equipped for dealing with an unexpected breech presentation. In this regard, the desire to increase safety by being proactive could be detrimental to the safety of some by de-skilling the providers of maternity care.

ANALYSIS AND PLACE OF BIRTH

In general, birth in hospital has been promoted as safer than birth at home. The tyranny of distance has had some influence on this view but in reality in most instances birth at home is safe. In a recent report on the outcomes for planned home births in Victoria in 2003, 90%

of women had a vaginal birth, regardless of where the birth took place (Bilcliff 2004). The rate of induction or augmentation of labour was 9% and the caesarean section rate 8%. These figures reflect world's best practice standards as set by the World Health Organization. Comparably, in the same year in Victoria, just 37% of women went into labour spontaneously and the overall caesarean rate for Victoria was 29%.

Comparing birth outcomes at home or in hospital is fraught with difficulty due to the relatively small numbers of women birthing at home, and the highly selective nature of the population. This can bias figures in both a positive and negative way.

RANZCOG has made a statement about home birth (2004) which says that:

Women seeking home birth should be informed regarding the increased risks of home birth in comparison to hospital birth for low risk women, as demonstrated by available evidence.

A further point is made that they should be 'counseled regarding the significance of these risks as applied to their own obstetric condition'.

The critical question in relation to homebirth for women who are truly low risk is the strength of the evidence, and the actual level of risk. The published evidence in the Australian setting relates to an increased risk of perinatal death, although the numbers in the two studies quoted are relatively small (Sullivan 1999, Bastion et al 1998). There have been some examples of successful midwifery-led homebirth programmes funded by two state governments (Western Australia and South Australia). What is lacking from the published evidence is an accurate assessment of risk for low risk women, who have been properly screened and counselled, and who choose to give birth with an experienced midwife who is able to arrange timely transfer should problems arise. Until such evidence is available from studies using appropriately rigorous methodology, it is hard to justify the RANZCOG statement as the 'increased risk' cannot be quantified.

References

Australian Bureau of Statistics Census 2001. Australian Government, Canberra

Australian College of Midwives 2003 National Guidelines for Consultation and Referral. Australian College of Midwives, Canberra

Australian College of Midwives 2005 Philosophy statement. Online. Available: http://www.acmi.org.au/text/corporate_documents/position/Philosophy.doc

Bastian H 2003 Variations in perceptions of risk between doctors and patients: risks look different when they are closer to home. Australian Prescriber (26)1: 20–21

Bastion H, Kierse MJ, Lancaster PA 1998 Perinatal death associated with planned home birth in Australia: population based study. British Medical Journal 317(7155): 384–388

Bilcliff A 2004 Outcomes for planned homebirths in Victoria. Birth Matters 8(4): 15

Buist R, Cahill A 2004 Benchmarking in obstetrics 2000–2003. Women's Hospitals Australasia, Canberra

Clarke R 2004 Health care and notions of risk. Therapeutic guidelines, Melbourne

Department of Health NSW 1989 Maternity services in New South Wales. Final Report of the Ministerial Taskforce on Obstetric Services in New South Wales. Department of Health, Sydney

Department of Human Services 2004 Having a baby in Victoria. Online. Available: www.health.viv.gov.au/maternity/models/index.htm

Hannah ME, Hannah WJ, Hewson SA et al 2000. Planned caesarean section versus planned vaginal birth for breech presentation at term: a randomized multi-centre trial. Lancet 356: 1375–1385

Health Department Victoria 1990 Having a baby in Victoria. Final Report of the Ministerial Review into Birthing Services in Victoria. Health Department Victoria, Melbourne

Heaman M, Beaton J, Gupton A, Sloan J 1992 A comparison of childbirth expectations in high-risk and low-risk pregnant women. Clinical Nursing Research 1(3): 252–265

Heaman M, Gupton A, Gregory D 2004 Factors influencing pregnant women's perceptions of risk. Maternal Child Nursing 29(2): 111–116

Kelly J 2004 Maternity revamp sparks baby fears, Herald Sun, 22 Jun. Online. Available: www.heraldsun.news.com.au/printpage/0,5481,9918332,00.html 20 Aug 2004

Kildea S 2001 Birthing in the Bush – Maternity services in remote areas of Australia. Paper presented at the 19th National Annual Conference of the Council of Remote Area Nurses of Australia Conference – From generalist to specialist, 28–31 Aug. The Australian Remote Area Nurse, Cairns

Kildea S, Wardaguga M, Dawumal M 2004 Maningrida women. Birthing business in the Bush. Liquid Rain Design. Online. Available: www.maningrida.com/mac/bwc/birthing/index.html

Kotaska A 2004 Inappropriate use of randomized controlled trials to evaluate complex phenomena: case study of vaginal breech delivery. British Medical Journal 329(7473): 1030–1042

Laws P, Sullivan EA 2004 Australia's mothers and babies 2002. Australian Institute of Health and Welfare, Canberra. Online. Available: www.npsu.unsw.edu.au/ps13high.htm

McGeary K 1994 The influence of guarding on the developing mother–unborn child relationship. In: Field PA, Marck PB (eds) Uncertain motherhood: negotiating the risks of the childbearing years. Sage Publications, London

McPhee J 2002 Perceptions of risk – a legal perspective. Australian Prescriber 25(5): 114–115

Molloy D 2004 Caesarean section: the end point in reproductive emancipation for women? RANZCOG Obstetrics and Gynaecology Magazine 6(3): 187–188

Nassar N, Roberts C, Barratt A et al on behalf of the Decision Aid for presentation trial collaborators (in press) Evaluation of a decision aid for women with breech presentation at term: a randomised trial. British Journal of Obstetrics and Gynaecology

National Aboriginal and Torres Strait Islander Health Council 2001 National Aboriginal and Torres Strait Islander Health Strategy. NATSIHC, Canberra

National Health and Medical Research Council 1996 Options for effective care in childbirth. Australian Government Printing Service, Canberra

National Health and Medical Research Council 1998 Review of services offered by midwives. Australian Government Printing Service, Canberra

Northern Territory Department of Health and Community Services 1992 Review of birthing services in the Northern Territory of Australia. Australian Government Printing Service, Darwin

Private Health Insurance Administration Council 2005 Industry statistics. Online. Available: http://www.phiac.gov.au/statistics/index.htm

RANZCOG 2004 Home births, College Statement No 2. RANZCOG, Melbourne

RANZCOG 2005 Breech deliveries at term, College Statement No 11. RANZCOG, Melbourne. Online. Available: www.ranzcog.edu.au

Reiger K 2000 Telling tales: health professionals' and mothers' constructions of 'choice' in childbirth. Sociological Sites/Sights, TASA Conference, Flinders University, Adelaide, 6–7 Dec

Reiger K 2003 Difficult labour: struggles to change Australian maternity care. Australian Midwifery Action Research Project Vol 2. Centre for Family Health and Midwifery, University of Sydney, Sydney

Roberts C, Tracy S, Peat B 2000 Rates for obstetric intervention among private and public patients in Australia: population based descriptive study. British Medical Journal 321(7245): 137–141

Robson S, Ellwood D 2003 Should obstetricians support a 'term cephalic trial'? Australian and New Zealand Journal of Obstetrics and Gynaecology 43: 341–343

Senate Community Affairs Reference Committee 1999 Rocking the cradle. A report into childbirth procedures. Commonwealth of Australia, Canberra

Slovic P 1999 Trust, emotion, sex, politics and science: surveying the risk assessment battlefield. Risk Analysis 19(4): 689–701

Sullivan P 1999 Perinatal death associated with planned homebirth in Australia. Home births are not justified in Australia. British Medical Journal 318(7183): 605–606

Swan N 2005 Evidence-based journalism: a forlorn hope. Medical Journal of Australia 183(4): 194–195

Trudgen R 2000 Why warriors lie down and die. Aboriginal Resources Development, Darwin

WA Legislative Assembly Select Committee 1995 Report on Intervention in Childbirth. Government of Western Australian, Perth

Wardaguga M 2004. In: Kildea S, Wardaguga M, Dawumal M Maningrida women. Birthing business in the Bush. Liquid Rain Design. Online. Available www.maningrida.com/mac/bwc/birthing/index.html

Willis E 1989 Medical dominance. Allen and Unwin, Sydney

Wilson J 1994 Quality in clinical healthcare risk modification. Health Business Summary, Apr

World Health Organization 1998 Every pregnancy faces risk. Division of Reproductive Health, WHO, Geneva. Online. Available: http://www.who.int/docstore/world-health-day/en/pages1998/whd98_05.html

Chapter **12**

Choices, Collaboration and Outcomes in Australia

Jennifer Cameron and David Ellwood

INTRODUCTION

This chapter will explore: factors governing choice; how choices are made; processes for resolving conflict; use of reflection and the future of maternity choices in Australia.

Various factors influence choice in maternity care in Australia. Geographical region is a major influence, with limited choices available in the rural regions and even less in remote areas. This is because these areas are relatively sparsely populated. The majority of Australians live in the capital cities, most of which are coastal (see Figure 11.1, Chapter 11).

CHOICE IN RURAL AND REMOTE AREAS

Rural and remote areas are often inaccessible at certain times of the year. In Northern Australia roads may be impassable for months at a time in the wet season; airstrips may be under water or inaccessible due to stormy weather. In a 1999 study most stakeholders agreed that it would be beneficial for primigravidae and women with a high risk condition to continue to be transferred to a regional centre to birth (Kildea 1999). However, the majority of indigenous women felt that it would be safe for healthy multiparas to birth in their remote community. Although it was agreed that it was safer for primigravidae and women with high risk conditions to birth in the regional centre, this was not without its problems. Women reported they get 'humbug from drunks and relatives' who take their money and leave them with none (Kildea 1999) ('humbug' is an indigenous saying that refers to harassing or nagging from another person). In indigenous culture if a family member asks for money (or goods) then you give it. It is a very communal and sharing culture. No money means little food and as the women are transferred in the last month of pregnancy, this leaves them vulnerable to the effects of poor nutrition, most particularly anaemia with its attendant risks to the mother and her unborn baby. Thermo-protective brown fat is laid down in the last months of pregnancy, and loss of this important resource may result in low birth weight and a poor transition to extrauterine life. There is also an established link between low birth weight and chronic diseases in childhood for indigenous children, so pregnancy outcome and child health are directly linked (Kildea 1999).

SERVICE PROVISION

Many rural birthing units in Australia have been closed – at least 40 in recent years (Hirst 2005, Tracy 2005, Vernon 2004). Many have closed in response to shortages of general practitioners who practise obstetrics, and shortages of midwives; but some have closed due to the mistaken belief that it is safer for women to birth in larger centres. In theory, this may sound sensible but in reality it means women have to travel long distances to give birth. Birthing a baby in a small rural unit with a midwife or general practitioner in attendance is likely to be far safer than birthing a baby in a car on the side of the highway as has happened recently. As reported by the Sydney Sun-Herald:

> A publican's wife in a tiny township had to deliver a baby on a car seat after the young mother had covered only one-third of a 165 kilometer road trip trying to get to a regional hospital.

> (Gregory 2005)

Shortages of general practitioners who practise obstetrics have mainly resulted from the social and emotional costs of operating as a sole practitioner, although fear of litigation and costs of indemnity insurance are also given as reasons. Rural and remote areas have trouble attracting and retaining skilled staff, both medical and midwifery (AMWAC 1998, Kildea 2001, Mohen 2004, Vernon 2004). Some units have closed because they do not have the capabilities for caesarean section, although many units are close enough to a regional centre to allow safe transport should transfer become necessary. Closure of these units limits choice for the women in those communities who now have to travel to larger centres for their care. From one perspective they may have more choice in terms of birth interventions and pain management options but is this useful when all medical procedures carry risks? As well, dislocation from their family, particularly other children, may have detrimental consequences on family relationships. One family chose to birth at home rather than travel to the nearest large centre for the birth of their third child. The birth was easy and trouble-free in contrast to the:

> . . . stress and heart-searching the family went through during the pregnancy as they sought safe maternity care that was acceptable to them . . .

> (Robotham 2004)

The family wished to birth with a midwife as their primary carer but the model was unavailable at the large centre at the time Mrs F. booked in:

> As the birth approached she felt increasingly unhappy about the prospect of giving birth in a medical environment under the care of strangers. The couple decided they would stay at home.

> (Robotham 2004)

As noted by a leading Australian midwife academic, Associate Professor Sally Tracy, this case was:

> . . . an absolute indictment of our maternity services in Australia, where women really don't have a choice . . .

> (Robotham 2004)

Indigenous women and their families are those most affected by the requirement to transfer out of their community to a larger centre to give birth as the majority of women who live in remote and rural areas of Australia are indigenous.

INSURANCE ISSUES

Women with private health insurance appear to have more birthing options than those women using the public hospital system. However, as noted by Roberts et al (2000) women using the private health system experienced a higher rate of intervention compared to their public hospital counterparts. Of all primiparas at low risk of complications in private hospitals 18% achieved a non-interventionist spontaneous vaginal birth compared with 28% of private patients in a public hospital and 39% of public patients. Among private patients with an epidural the most likely outcome was an instrumental delivery with an episiotomy. Among similar public patients the most likely outcome was a vaginal birth without an episiotomy (Roberts et al 2000).

It has been argued that the increased rate of intervention in the women accessing private hospital care may be due to this group being generally older than those in public hospitals and therefore at higher risk of complications (Roff 2004). However, the fact that public hospitals house the tertiary perinatal centres dealing with high risk patients would imply that they should have higher rates of intervention, which is not the case. This suggests that there may be an element of choice by the obstetrician or the woman in some of the interventions in private hospitals. Women accessing public hospital care are likely to have more models of care from which to choose but this does not always equate to quality of care. In the Victorian review of birthing services (Health Department Victoria 1990), women using the services of a privately practising obstetrician were those most satisfied with their care episode. It can be argued that this satisfaction is due to continuity of carer and consistency of information rather that the obstetric model per se. Perhaps women may be prepared

to sacrifice a higher intervention rate for the advantage of continuity of care.

CHOICE AND TERTIARY CENTRES

Tertiary perinatal centres are likely to offer more models of care; this however, does not always result in a better quality of care for women. Team midwifery and shared care models often result in the woman being exposed to many different people during her episode of care. This has resulted in dissatisfaction with maternity care (Brown et al 2001). Care with a known, primary midwife has proven popular and safe for Australian women. In a recent report (Women's and Children's Hospital, Adelaide 2005), favorable outcomes were achieved by women using the publicly funded group midwifery practice when compared with the State average. In this model the woman has continuity of carer and a back-up midwife. Satisfaction with care was not measured in this report.

There are examples from tertiary centres in which midwifery care and high risk pregnancy management is a collaborative venture. More research needs to be done to better understand how this kind of care model can improve outcomes for high risk women.

RESEARCH, EVIDENCE AND CHOICE

A future research study to be carried out in Australia has the potential to affect choice and increase risk for women. The ACTOBAC trial (A Collaborative Trial of Birth After Caesarean) is a randomised controlled trial that compares a policy of vaginal birth with that of elective repeat caesarean section for women at term who have had a previous caesarean section. Participants for this trial will be sought from Australia, New Zealand and possibly Canada. As one consumer group, Maternity Coalition, state, 'there is great concern from consumers, midwives, obstetricians and academics alike that this trial is unethical and will have a huge impact on women's choice and care in the future' (Caines 2003). Participating women will be randomised to caesarean section with its slightly increased risk of maternal death (albeit infinitesimal) and increased morbidity; the increased risk of placenta praevia and placenta accreta in future pregnancies (Tippet 2004, Usta et al 2005). As well there are long-term risks such as adhesion formation that may increase the rate of ectopic pregnancy and of small bowel obstruction (Bernstein 2005).

Vaginal birth after previous caesarean (VBAC) is an issue about which many Australian women need to make a decision. Issues for women include the place of birth, pain management and how much intervention they will have, such as electronic fetal monitoring and intravenous access. Women are generally counselled about the 0.5–1% risk of scar rupture during labour and are recommended to have continuous electronic fetal monitoring as fetal heart rate changes are an early sign of scar dehiscence. Most centres also recommend intravenous access and birth in a standard birth room in a tertiary centre. This is in contrast to what many women want, which is their VBAC experience to be as natural as possible, and some request to birth in a family birth centre or at home. This is often in response to a traumatic first birth that led to the primary caesarean.

Caesarean Awareness Recovery Education Support South Australia (CARESSA) is a community based organisation of women whose primary focus is to support women healing from a previous traumatic or upsetting birth experience by caesarean. Women meet and discuss their experiences. The following are some of the comments (from the CARESSA website) made by these women as to why they would choose a VBAC:

Because it is the one thing that will give me back my life, erase the feelings of abject failure and make me feel like a true mother, not one that can't even accomplish the first task required of her, that is giving birth to her child . . .

I had always wanted a natural birth and was so disappointed and upset by the caesarean. Birth is an essential experience, a woman's rite of passage . . .

For me it is about following a path that millions of women have followed, nature has always planned for the majority of women to birth vaginally . . .

Because just like any other woman, I have the ability and the right to birth my baby as nature intended . . .

After a traumatic birth many women wish for a better sense of control of their next birth experience. Home or the birth centre may appeal to them as safer alternatives – safe from the intervention that they dread. Given that the rate of lower segment scar rupture in those women experiencing spontaneous onset of labour is 0.5%, this would seem to be the case. When Syntocinon is used to induce labour where there is a scar in the uterus, the rate of scar rupture rises to 5%.

How women perceive the risk of VBAC is likely to depend on the counsellor and the way in which risks are presented. For some women a 1 in 200 risk of scar rupture may well be an acceptable risk, as long as they are aware of the factors which may increase their risk. Absolute risk of any outcome needs to be framed in the context of how this compares with other birth choices. However, using relative risk without informing a woman about the absolute risk can be very misleading.

How choices are enacted in one pregnancy can influence future pregnancies. In the following illustration Susan (pseudonym) was directed to push by her caregivers with serious consequences:

At about 4.30 I yelled that I needed to push. The midwives told me that I couldn't push, to use the gas and breathe through that urge and that the doctor was on the way. Well – the doctor looked inside and said 'yep, she is ready to go'; 10 cm dilated and that baby's head was waiting to come out. So then the push started . . . I pushed five times, each time moving her slowly further down. The midwives told me to change my way of pushing. I put my feet on their hips, grabbed hold of my thighs near my knees, stuck my chin down to my chest . . . I pushed so hard that her head was birthed and on the next breath her body followed. She was born with her right hand beside her head, near her ear. I sustained a 4th degree tear. I guess that if I could have changed anything, it would have been to not be on my back and to have controlled my pushing a bit more . . .

The prognosis after this birth was that for any subsequent pregnancies caesarean section was recommended due to the possibility of another fourth-degree tear. Susan was told this could possibly lead to total bowel incontinence requiring a colostomy bag. As Susan explains

I could not believe this. I researched why I tore, I researched the exact numbers and statistics linked to my situation. The more I read I was not convinced that major abdominal surgery was equal to the small risk involved in a vaginal birth, for me and my body.

On presentation for her second pregnancy Susan was again advised to have an elective caesarean section by all but one obstetrician whom she spoke to, with no advice on how to achieve vaginal birth with minimal risk of tearing. She also declined active management of third stage and was told by her obstetrician:

Sure it's all lovely and good to deliver the placenta naturally, but it isn't very nice to die naturally of massive blood loss from a postpartum haemorrhage.

Nathan was born after a 2-hour labour, birth weight 3820 g; Susan required two sutures to a small second-degree perineal tear. And as for the third stage:

I didn't have the syntometrine injection; the placenta was birthed naturally in its own time and with no problems. Nathan suckled a few times and his apgars were 9 at 1 min, 10 at 10 mins.

I laughed a lot after his birth; I felt and still feel so powerful. I birthed him with my body, no help, no drugs, minimal tearing. So take that evil doctor – I don't need a colostomy bag and I didn't die from a post-partum haemorrhage when I birthed the placenta. I am living proof that a woman who sustains a massive tear, can

birth again vaginally. It required a lot of reading and soul searching, and a major understanding of WHY the tear occurred in the first place.

Another woman exercised her right to choose a caesarean section because her obstetrician had said earlier in the antenatal period that she could have one. At the point of this story she is overdue and has fears about her baby's health:

The next morning I told my obstetrician that I wanted to have a caesarean. He did another internal and said he might be able to break my waters now, though he wasn't 100% sure. And I just said 'no thank you I've had enough of that'. My obstetrician had told me from day one that I could have a caesarean if I wanted to. Now I'd decided to have one he was all funny about it and they were quite nasty about having to fit me in, which made me feel like I was being a burden on them. Most of them I trusted a lot over myself but when they kept trying to induce me despite the heart rate, I didn't [trust them]. And when my obstetrician wouldn't listen to me and said 'no' to a caesarean I knew they never really trusted me. He made me feel like I had no control over anything but at the end of the day it was my decision and I got my caesarean.

I didn't know there were any risks to having a caesar apart from infection; I wouldn't know any risks even now. He told me that having a caesar may mean I wouldn't be able to have a natural birth next time and little things like that. And he said I could still wear bikinis because the scar is covered. But no one said anything about any risks to my baby, I was wondering about how they got the fluid out of his lungs.

(Parratt 2005)

Risk presentation is an issue for all maternity care providers. It is essential to ensure that women are given adequate and clear information on which to make an informed choice about their childbirth experience. The amount of information a woman has to enable her to make her decision will influence the available choices. Most women choose caesarean section because of the perceived better outcome for the baby. Most women do not realise that caesarean section carries an increased morbidity for both mother and baby. According to Tippett (2004) current evidence suggests that elective caesarean birth is not associated with a measurable increase in maternal mortality but the data are less reassuring with respect to maternal morbidity. Tippett (2004) also highlights the lack of evidence supporting caesarean birth as neuroprotective for the fetus; as well, in spite of increasing rates of caesarean birth, there has been no decline in nerve palsies or fractures. Pre-labour caesarean is also associated with an increase in central nervous system depression, feeding difficulties, and respiratory distress, although the latter declines markedly with gestation close to 40 weeks (Tippet 2004).

LEGAL INFLUENCES

Laws will influence choice for women. In Australia recently a woman was reported to child protection authorities after she failed to turn up for antenatal visits and exercised her right to choose her mode of birth. Ms Smith (pseudonym) was booked for a repeat caesarean section following two previous caesareans. She chose to birth vaginally in a regional hospital, not the major metropolitan centre she had originally booked into. The birth was normal and uneventful. Currently in Australia the fetus has no legal rights and the right to withhold consent to treatment is a fundamental common-law right of all patients (Staunton & Chiarella 2003). The medical response to this story took the perspective of what this woman had 'got away with' as contrasted with the Australian College of Midwives:

Every woman has the right to choose her caregiver and place of birth. The decision by Ms Smith to change from one hospital to another for her antenatal and intrapartum care is her right.

Argument from the Queensland AMA that Ms Smith put her baby at risk by changing from one hospital to another are not supported

by evidence and amount to a serious and unsubstantiated allegation that obstetric and midwifery staff at the alternative hospital were negligent in their provision of care to Ms Smith.

Caesarean section carries increased risks of mortality and morbidity for both mother and baby and is not a procedure that should be being routinely undertaken.

(Vernon 2005)

In this instance the Australian laws governing the mandatory reporting of potential child abuse were used by hospital staff to try to force the woman to undergo a repeat caesarean section against her will.

The philosophy of a professional body will also affect the way in which its members interact and communicate with other members of the healthcare team, as the next section illustrates.

COLLABORATION

The way in which midwives and doctors relate to each other influences choice and outcomes for women. The following story, told by a midwife in a Victorian provincial city, illustrates the way tensions are sometimes resolved in the public hospital sector where obstetrics is usually given more authority than midwifery and lip service is paid to woman-centred care. For confidentiality reasons the midwife remains anonymous:

'We need to know if she is fully dilated' yelled the Resident Medical Officer (RMO) who was red-faced with agitation. Seeing a woman push **without our permission** *was not an option. 'We need to know if she can push.' (original emphasis)*

(Anon 2004)

The midwife caring for the woman was aware that she felt like pushing and had encouraged her to 'breathe through' the contractions until she couldn't suppress the urge to push. The fetal heart rate was satisfactory. At this point the RMO returned to the room and would not allow the woman to push unless authorised by a medical professional following confirmation of full dilatation. The midwifery philosophy of working with the woman, based on trust of women's bodies, was overridden by the power given by institutions to medical practitioners, experienced or otherwise. The RMO performed the vaginal examination, announced that full dilatation had been reached and declared, 'You can push now' (Anon 2004).

Scenes such as the above are played out daily in many hospitals in Australia. A recent report into birth centre services in Queensland found evidence of poor communication and lack of collegiality between the birth centre midwives and obstetricians; and also between birth centre midwives and midwives working in the standard maternity care wards (Nicholl & McCann 2005). This demonstrates the effect of philosophy on professional relationships. The birth centre midwives probably held a different belief about birthing than their midwife and obstetric colleagues. The report stated that the relationship between the birth centre midwives and the obstetricians was characterised by mistrust and lack of respect (Nicholl & McCann 2005). Exceptions exist such as Nambour Private Hospital in Queensland where the care is based on women's needs and not on hospital routines or doctor/midwife preferences (Staff 2000). However, the art of midwifery often struggles beneath the weight of the medical model as Aicken (1999) states:

> The art of midwifery does exist within the hospital birthing environment. Albeit of a silent nature.

Collaboration between women and midwives does not always happen appropriately. Knowledge of cultural mores and local customs is essential before embarking on a new course of action. In one remote area a new midwife in an indigenous community decided it might be a good idea to start antenatal classes once a week. She went and spoke to non-indigenous community women and set the classes up for a Thursday. No one turned up to the classes. The midwife had failed to talk to the indigenous community members before commencing the new programme. The indigenous women in this community did not like to come together in the manner that had been set up. In addition, Thursday was payday and there were other more important activities in process. Failing to communicate appropriately affected choice for the women in the community. Having the classes on a Thursday and in the current format meant they could not attend and therefore missed out on important information (Kildea & Wardaguga 2004).

In collaborating with women, midwives work alongside the woman and follow her lead. It is the role of the midwife to provide the information to enable women to make an informed choice.

OUTCOMES: REFLECTIONS

Reflection is now widely used in the Australian healthcare field by medical professionals and midwives. As a formal process reflective practice forms part of educational curricula for midwives and medical practitioners. Reflection on outcomes in obstetric departments has usually been restricted to examining serious adverse outcomes such as perinatal mortality. However, in recent times it has become more common to conduct regular clinical audit, with reflection on both good and bad outcomes as well as interventions. An example of this occurs at The Canberra Hospital, where each week a multiprofessional meeting takes place at which midwives (both labour ward and birth centre-based), registrars and specialists discuss each birth for the last week. This is an opportunity for all to reflect on outcomes, and discuss how these might be improved. This reflective audit process has now been extended to many of the regional centres which feed in to Canberra, including a number of the smaller general practitioner- and midwife-led units. Perhaps consideration should be given to inviting consumers of the maternity services to these meetings!

FACTORS CONSTRAINING THE USE OF REFLECTION

According to Taylor (2000: 121), not enough time is the most common excuse for Australian midwives not incorporating reflection into their working lives. However, personal reflection can take place anywhere at any time. Certainly, it can be difficult or simply impossible to leave a busy clinical area to attend a clinical audit meeting, even if the meeting is right next door. Scheduling these meetings regularly and frequently improves the likelihood of all staff being able to attend some meetings over the year.

Inappropriate application of the principles of clinical risk management may also influence willingness to reflect by healthcare professionals. Insistence on rigid adherence to guidelines by senior hospital staff and punitive actions by administrators towards mistakes may inhibit reflective processes, encourage 'robotic' actions and thus diminish clinical judgment. The ability to think critically is very important to safe practice which is why this topic has been incorporated into medical and midwifery curricula.

Just as women are encouraged to write a birth plan, so they are also encouraged to reflect on their birth experience Women have traditionally reflected on their personal experiences of birth. Stories are exchanged and comparisons drawn. This ritualistic type of behaviour probably assists each woman to incorporate the childbearing experience into her life. In 21st-century Australia busy lifestyles often do not allow this reflective exchange to take place and sometimes the only opportunity a woman has for recounting a previous birth is to her carer when booking in for the next birth. This has the potential to limit choices for women as time constraints may affect the quality of this exchange. Encouraging women to reflect on their birthing experience while still under the care of the midwife, general practitioner or obstetrician may reduce this possibility.

WHAT DOES THE FUTURE HOLD FOR AUSTRALIAN FAMILIES?

Exciting changes are happening all over Australia in relation to maternity services. The many birthing services reviews and the sustained efforts of lobby groups have resulted in most State governments rebuilding, or agreeing to rebuild, their maternity services. Pressure is still being exerted on the Federal government to make changes to the national health insurance system, Medicare, to enable Australian families to claim the cost of private midwifery care. Collaborative models where maternity care is shared between the obstetrician and the midwife are being encouraged; these collaborative arrangements are seen to be of particular benefit to women with high risk pregnancies who ordinarily would find it difficult to access midwifery care. Additionally, in some areas, women do have the choice of a midwife as their primary carer. Midwifery education has changed with a Bachelor of Midwifery degree available as entry to practice, as well as the traditional postgraduate (nursing) midwifery course.

Opportunities for women to become more involved in determining options for maternity care are increasing, with more consumer involvement on health service committees, better systems of complaints management and more quality internet consumer information health sites, such as the Australasian Cochrane Collaboration.

SUMMARY

Risk and choice in maternity services in Australia are governed by many factors, not the least of which is the multicultural nature of the population and the vast distances that lie between the populations. The nature of Australian maternity services is currently in a state of flux, with expanding options for choice of primary caregiver. There is still a lot of work to do to ensure culturally and physically safe and acceptable services in the rural and remote areas but the work has begun. The dedicated efforts of various community groups and individuals have at last begun to bear fruit and Australian society will be the healthier for it.

References

Aicken N 1999 Hear ye the silent voice: narratives in the art of midwifery. Masters thesis (unpublished). Used with permission

AMWAC (Australian Medical Workforce Advisory Committee) 1998 Influences on participation in the Australian Medical Workforce. AMWAC Report No 4. Australian Government Printer, Sydney

Anonymous 2004 A brilliant birth. Birth Matters 8(1): 10–12

Bernstein P 2005 Complications of caesarean deliveries, clinical update. CME programs, Medscape Ob/Gyn and Womens Health. Online. Available: www.medscape.com Sep 2005

Brown S, Bruinsma F, Darcy MA, Lumley J 2001 Victorian survey of recent mothers 2000 Report 1. Women's views and experiences of maternity care. Department of Human Services, Centre for the Study of Mothers' and Children's Health, Melbourne

Caines J 2003 ACTOBAC. Birth Matters, Journal of Maternity Coalition 7(7): 3

CARESSA Online. Available: http://homepages.picknowl.com.au/caressa/

Gregory D 2005 Delivery van: Kharlie's long drive to give birth, Sydney Sun-Herald, May 1. Online. Available: www.smh.com.au/news/National/Delivery-van-Kharlies-long-drive-to-give-birth 2 May 2005

Health Department Victoria 1990 Having a baby in Victoria, Final Report of the Ministerial Review into Birthing Services in Victoria. Health Department Victoria, Melbourne

Hirst C 2005 Re-birthing. Report of the Review of Maternity Services in Queensland, Queensland Health Department, Queensland

Kildea S 1999 And the women said . . ., Report on Birthing Services for Aboriginal Women from Remote Top End Communities. Territory Health Service, Darwin

Kildea S 2001 Birthing in the Bush – Maternity services in remote areas of Australia. Paper presented at the 19th National Annual Conference of the Council of Remote Area Nurses of Australia Conference – From generalist to specialist, 28–31 Aug. The Australian Remote Area Nurse, Cairns

Kildea S, Wardaguga M, Dawumal M 2004 Maningrida women. Birthing business in the Bush. Liquid Rain Design. Online. Available: http://www.maningrida.com/mac/bwc/bush.html

Mohen D 2004 The future of obstetric practice in provincial Australia. RANZCOG Obsterics and Gynaecology Magazine 6(1): 10–11

Nicholl M, McCann Y 2005 Review of birth centre services. Queensland Government, Queensland Health, Royal Brisbane and Women's Hospital, Brisbane

Parratt J 2005 Unpublished PhD, work in progress

Roberts C, Tracy S, Peat B 2000 Rates for obstetric intervention among private and public patients in Australia: population based descriptive study. British Medical Journal 321(7245): 137–141

Robotham J 2004 Hard labour: a family's search for maternity care. Sydney Morning Herald, 14 Oct. Online. Available: www.smh.com.au. Reproduced with permission

Roff M 2004 AHA pushing misinformation based on 'half-baked' study. Australian Private Hospitals Association, media release. Online. Available: http://www.apha.org.au/read/2394521048.html Apr 14 2004

Staff L 2000 Enriching care. The Selangor Maternity Care Experience. Online. Available: www.acegraphics.com.au/articles/staff01.html

Staunton P, Chiarella M 2003 Nursing and the law, 5th edn. Churchill Livingstone, Sydney, ch 4

Taylor B 2000 Reflective practice: a guide for nurses and midwives. Allen and Unwin, Sydney

Tippet C 2004 Primary elective caesarean section: patient's choice or obstetrician's dilemma. Obstetrics and Gynaecology 6(3): 18–19

Tracy S 2005 It's happening – midwifery led maternity services at last! Future Birth: With Woman With Child, Lecture Tour. Birth International. Online. Available: www. acegraphics.com.au/articles/sally02.html Nov 2005

Usta IM, Hobeika EM, Musa AA et al 2005 Placenta previa-accreta: risk factors and complications. American Journal of Obstetrics and Gynaecology 193(3) Pt 2: 1045–1049

Vernon B 2004 Birth in the Bush – a dying art. Media release, Australian College of Midwives and the Council for Remote Area Nurses. Online. Available: www.acmi.org.au/ Apr 2004

Vernon B 2005 Advocacy update, Midwifery E-Bulletin, Feb. Online. Available: www.acmi.org.au/bulletin.htm

Women and Children's Hospital, Adelaide 2005 First Highlights Report. Central Information Services (CIS) statistical data collection Jan 2004–Mar 2005. WCH, Adelaide

Chapter 13

Risk and Choice: a US Midwifery Perspective

Janet Brooks

INTRODUCTION

Over time, as a midwife, I have discovered a universal thread in women who are expecting a baby. All want a healthy baby. Planned pregnancy or not, a healthy baby is the driving force for the next several months. Of course, no one would want anything other than a healthy baby. It is not that anyone would not want a healthy baby – the issue in question is how to go about having a healthy baby. The perception of how to have a problem-free pregnancy, and therefore a healthy baby, and what is risk, and what is not, is as different as each individual mother. Communicating about and understanding pregnancy and the birth process is what midwives do and try to do in a climate of confidence rather than a climate of doubt. This is often undermined by the over-medicalisation of pregnancy care (Rothman 1991, Wagner 1994), where a woman's risk status does not necessarily determine the level of care she receives (Dobie et al 1994, Haire & Elsberry 1991, Oakley et al 1996).

Many studies[1] have shown that care given by Certified Nurse Midwives (CNMs) is as effective or more effective as that by a physician for

---

[1] These studies include Bell & Mill 1989, Dobie et al 1994, Dower & Miller 1999, Gabay & Wolfe 1995, 1997, Greulich et al 1994, Haire & Elsberry 1991, Law & Lam 1999, MacDorman & Singh 1998, Oakley et al 1996, Rosen & Hobel 1986, Schlenzka 1999, State of Washington 1988.

an uncomplicated pregnancy. The midwifery model of care stresses fewer medical interventions, and less use of technology and results in birth and overall health outcomes equal to or better than those in obstetrical care, as well as producing significant savings to the healthcare systems in which they work (Rosen & Hobel 1986, Schlenzka 1999, State of Washington 1988). CNMs are cost effective without compromising the quality of care, spending more time with the client and discussing psychosocial aspects as well as evaluating the physiological changes.

A PIECE OF US MIDWIFERY HISTORY

Home births were the norm during the early 1900s in the USA, as in much of the world. Around the same time the US Federal Children's Bureau concluded a study on the health of American mothers and babies showing maternal and infant mortality rates higher than in several western European countries. In 1911 the New York City Commissioner of Health stated that the US

> is the only civilized country in the world in which the health as well as the life and future wellbeing of mothers and infants is not safeguarded so far as possible through the training and control of midwives.
>
> (Rooks 1997)

This same year the first midwifery programme was opened at Bellevue Hospital in New York City (Speert 1980). Through the next 20 years or so the emerging idea of prenatal care became intertwined with public health nurses and 'granny midwives' coordinating care for pregnant women. Nurses who were also trained as midwives seemed to be the answer. Nurse-midwives (a new term coined by Dr Frederick Taussig, a St Louis physician) came into being (Rooks 1997).

This resulted in the establishment of the Frontier Nursing Service in 1925 in Hyden, Kentucky by Mary Breckinridge, an American nurse and British trained midwife who felt the combination of nursing and a separate midwifery training would best serve women and their families. She recruited several British midwives to help her get started. For the first 25–30 years home births were the norm, but the national trend towards hospital birth rapidly advanced, and by 1975, 99% of all births took place in a hospital (National Center for Health Statistics 2005).

In the first half of the 20th century, most pregnancy care in the USA was by an obstetrician/ gynaecologist or a general practitioner, now known as primary care providers. The general public depends on professionals for advice, expertise and information for which they have been trained. Midwives, trained as experts to attend women in childbirth, were not seen as professionals, and even today, the perception is that midwives 'do it' in homes, and are not associated with the medical profession (personal experience and personal communications).

In this time period, education in anatomy and physiology and health, was generally very basic and most people were ignorant of how the body functioned. This was compounded by the 'birds and bees' approach when discussing human sexuality with adolescents. Litigation was not yet commonplace. The specialties of perinatology and maternal fetal medicine had not yet developed on a national level. In the period from 1900 to the 1960s, ultrasound was a rare event and a burgeoning science. Perinatal referral systems were not organised or well established in urban areas and non-existent in rural areas. Breastfeeding was shunned in favour of the newer and more 'scientifically' produced infant formulas. Midwives were scattered here and there, either in small home birth practices or in large medical centres. A few birth centres existed (Rooks 1997).

In 1955, Columbia University in New York City, in conjunction with the University Departments of Public Health and Nursing, the Maternity Center Association (MCA) and Kings County Hospital in Brooklyn, began the first nurse midwifery programme to provide clinical training in its academic medical centre. This same year the American College of Nurse-Midwifery was formed and its first meeting was held in 1956. The first issue of the *Nurse Midwife Bulletin* was published in December 1955 and this has now become a respected peer reviewed journal, the *Journal of Midwifery and Women's Health*.

Social movements of the 1960s included the Vietnam antiwar movement, the violent and still continuing civil rights movement, and the 'back-to-the-land' consumer movement. At the same time, the women's movement was spreading and 'the Pill' was introduced in 1960 (Rooks 1997).

This social and cultural climate in the USA at this time contributed to the widespread questioning of obstetrical practices culminating in the 1978 hearings before the US Congress (US Senate Congressional Hearings 1978). The subsequent rise of the home birth movement was a logical outcome. Advocating breastfeeding, home birth, natural remedies and non-interventional care, as well as personal responsibility, this grassroots group was actually quite progressive in lobbying for individualised, non-interventional care during pregnancy. Their mantra was that babies should be born where they were conceived. Organisations such as NAPSAC (International Association of Parents and Professionals for Safe Alternatives in Childbirth) and HOME (HOmebirth and Midwifery IndependencE) formed and networked through conferences and mailings. They focused on personal responsibility for women's health, partnership between her and her care provider, and self-education facilitating informed responsible and safe choices. NAPSAC is now an international organisation, and Stewarts' hallmark book, *The Five Standards for Safe Child-bearing*, is as relevant today as it was in the 1970s, with few exceptions (www.NAPSAC.org).

There were other groups, none of which became mainstream, but do still exist and today are well regarded; La Leche League International (LLL) and International Cesarean Awareness Network (ICAN) are two that are outstanding and maintain a relationship with professional groups including the American College of Obstetrics and Gynecology (ACOG) and the American Association of Pediatrics

(AAP). The information promulgated by LLL and ICAN is evidence based and scientifically sound, yet advocates evaluations on an individual basis.

In direct contrast to this approach is the maternal risk assessment formula, firmly entrenched in our blossoming regionalised perinatal care system. In 1972 the Robert Wood Johnson Foundation spearheaded a national programme to test this new idea and it has been in use since then.[2] This approach is the one that many of us, both midwives and physicians, know and work within: there is a scoring system for low, moderate and high risk classification with a mechanism for referral if risk increases. However, risk assessment is not perfect; some women classified as low risk have bad outcomes and some classified as high risk go on to have normal labours and births, despite all the interventions they receive because of their high risk classification. This has resulted in some physicians practising as if all pregnant women were high risk until the pregnancy is over (Rooks 1997).

Obstetricians initially learn in medical school how to use the scientific method and then as their education progresses, the amount of information and responsibilities increases exponentially and thus the line between facts and belief becomes blurred (Goer 1995). As an obstetric resident[3] there is barely time to sleep, never mind think. Clinical practices with no scientific foundation are adopted, mainly because they seem to work most of the time; then they become the standard of care, handed down from senior clinicians to trusting juniors.

---

[2] In the USA each of the 50 states and several territories have different healthcare systems, based on national, state and local budgets, and complex political controls.

[3] Residency in Obstetrics is usually a 4-year period where 1st, 2nd, 3rd and 4th year residents rotate through the different areas: gynaecology, oncology, high risk obstetrics, labour and delivery, and other smaller specialties. The labour and delivery suites in most teaching hospitals are managed by a 1st year resident with a 4th year 'chief' and obstetrician attending on call as needed.

How this actually happens is a very complicated process; politics, economics and the purchase of birth technology influence policies and procedures without benefit of scientific evaluation. Much of what is adopted is based more on description than analysis (Wagner 1994). The most well known example is the instantaneous and universal adoption of Electronic Fetal Monitoring (EFM) technology (Sandmire 1990). The scientific evaluation came after and showed no benefit with the use of this technology, and in fact showed an increase in interventions such as caesarean section, forceps deliveries and vacuum extractions, with no decrease in morbidity or mortality.[4] In the past decade there has been a move towards Evidence Based Medicine (EBM) (or evidence based practice, as I prefer), which can be said to be the integration of the best research evidence with clinical expertise and patient values.

WHAT DO WE MEAN BY RISK?

Asked to describe what risk means, 100 people will give almost as many answers. In the Oxford English Dictionary, 10th Edition, the word risk is both a noun and a verb. The noun is:

1–a situation involving exposure to danger; the possibility that something unpleasant will happen; 2–a person or thing causing a risk or regarded in relation to risk: a fire risk.

The verb is:

1–expose to danger or loss; act in such a way to incur the risk of. –incur risk by engaging in an action.

Merriam Webster's *Thesaurus* has synonyms for both uses of the word, some of which may be the more familiar understandings. Noun – danger, hazard, peril, jeopardy, chance, fortune, luck, accident, exposure, liability, openness.

---

[4] Many studies have shown this including: Curzen et al 1984, Grant 1993, Rosen & Dickenson 1993, Rosen & Hobel 1986, Sandmire 1990, Sykes et al 1983, Thacker 1987, Van Tuinen & Wolfe 1992.

Verb – venture, hazard, chance, jeopardise, endanger, imperil, dare, brave face, defy, confront, encounter, meet.

Most people find it hard to differentiate between the risk of having a car accident and the risk of having a baby affected with Down's syndrome. The risks you take when playing poker cannot be used to explain the risks of having a postpartum haemorrhage. As risk can only be estimated, it can be said that it is the comparison of probabilities. So the challenge is to effectively translate population risk data into clinical risk information that can be easily assimilated by the relevant individual (Edwards & Prior 1997).

In the discipline of epidemiology risk is again explained differently, and it is this set of facts that we are concerned with when conveying risk concepts to the pregnant woman and her family. The term 'risk factor' is used when referring to a condition or a noninfectious disease state. Sometimes the term causation is used, which implies the cause, but cause is determined by studying the risk factors.

PERSONAL INFORMATION AND EXPERIENCE DEMOGRAPHICS

The following discussion concerns the situation in an inner city hospital, which is the regional perinatal referral centre for the New York Metropolitan area: this includes parts of New Jersey and Connecticut. Between 25 and 28 midwives work in the hospital.

The patient demographic is predominantly immigrant, dominated by unmarried, young women from the Dominican Republic. Most come specifically to have their baby in the USA, do not have family support here and mostly do not speak English. Many have not graduated from high school but know it is safer and better to have a baby in the USA with the added plus of free medical care and American citizenship for their child. The second largest group are second generation Dominicans who have grown up in the USA, are married or in stable relationships, and who speak both English and Spanish. Most have jobs and are seeking post-high school education and are generally established in their community. The third group is mixed. There are very economically unstable Mexicans who have crossed the border and made their way to New York, many with no reading and/or writing skills, and very little prior healthcare. Next is an increasingly large group of West Africans, also not formally educated and with little or no prior healthcare. These women, for the most part, speak only their native dialect.

The next small group consists of South and Central American women from Peru, Argentina, Colombia, El Salvador, Honduras and Guatemala. The other women who come to our clinic are from various countries in Eastern Europe. Many of these women are more formally educated and do speak some English. There are also some African American women and Nuyoricans (Puerto Rican women who live and work in New York).

Many of the midwives have learned to speak 'medical Spanish', enough to get through a pre-natal visit with some translation by an available Spanish speaking staff member if there is a difficult issue. There is also a translation service available by phone and dual headsets if an appointment with patient, provider and translator can be coordinated. This is very helpful if someone speaks an unusual language. Some midwives, including myself, speak fluent Spanish and can have a more nuanced and meaningful conversation. However, I know that I, and several of my colleagues never feel that we can fully explain an issue of risk well to women of different cultures. Their cultures define the 'risk' of something good or bad in the context of their home traditions, some of which are based on the very different health-care and social infrastructure of the society they grew up in.

HOW WOMEN PERCEIVE RISK IN AN URBAN TERTIARY CARE SETTING

It is important to understand how the client thinks about risk if you are a care provider who communicates risk information. A care provider is in a position of power and can influence a woman's perception of risk: a nurse, a mid-wife, nurse practitioner or physician, due to their perceived position of authority, may consciously or unconsciously convey their bias of a certain situation or test, not realising their influence. Another source of bias is the nursing and medical assistant staff, even the clerical staff; by virtue of working in a medical clinic, they are perceived by clients as having some knowledge. Many providers in both my own setting and other practices around the country have confided situations where office staff have commiserated with a woman's situation and offered their heartfelt advice to her. A common occurrence that is a good example is the returning patient who has an unplanned pregnancy. Some women have already decided to either keep the pregnancy or to terminate, and others are confused and come for guidance about what to do. They need factual information about their options depending on the stage of pregnancy in order to think about their individual situation. They are often distraught and emotionally affected by the hormonal shifts common in early pregnancy and the unexpected event. A care provider who does not feel comfortable with terminations, as well as one who does, may inadvertently allow their bias to be known with the wording that they use. Many women will ask, 'What would you do?' or 'What should I do?' It is a decision the woman, and possibly her family, will live with for the rest of her life, either way. Remaining neutral is essential to safe, respectful and professional care.

Communicating risk can be done with simple verbal expressions or visual aids such as diagrams, graphs and charts (Gates 2004). One instance is explaining a marginal or total placenta praevia. A diagram is so much more instructive. (A placenta praevia is one that can implant directly over the cervix or in varying degrees next to the cervix). This possibility of an adverse event that cannot be controlled increases the perceived severity of the risk in question (Adams & Smith 2001). Since people like to feel as if they exert some control over their lives, an event that cannot be controlled is often felt to become more controllable by the use of technology. Discussions with midwives from every corner of the USA report an almost universal belief by their clients that 'more is better' and women would want all available testing and technology to feel assured of a healthy baby. The belief is that a higher rate of testing will decrease their chance of a baby with any problems. Ultrasound scans are viewed as the gold standard for ensuring a healthy baby and many women expect several spaced sonograms to 'see if the baby is OK', despite explanations of the optimal times for dating and anatomical survey sonography. There is a phrase that midwives 'Listen to Women'; however, reminding women that they themselves are usually the best source of information to determine position and movement or changes in baby's behaviour is received with scepticism. It is almost as if some women are detached from the growing baby in their abdomen, and need someone to tell them what is happening inside them. This illustrates the belief that some women do not have self-confidence and trust medical authorities above themselves.

In his book, *Expecting Trouble, What Expectant Parents should Know about Prenatal Care in America*, Strong (2000: 1) says, 'the singular lesson I've learned from my experience is that most American women are unduly anxious about their chances of developing pregnancy complications and simultaneously overoptimistic about our ability to cure them.'

An example of a woman with a very different mindset is the 46-year-old woman, pregnant for the first time, introduced to me at a coffee shop by a mutual friend. She was excited as well as ambivalent, a normal state for women in early pregnancy. She lives in the suburbs but had been referred to a tertiary care centre because an early sonogram had 'detected something'. The subsequent Level 2 sonogram had indicated a significant congenital anomaly. Her obstetrician informed her that this was incompatible with life and she was advised to terminate the pregnancy. It was at this time that we met and talked for many hours about what to do, what not to do and what it all meant. She was agonising because she felt this might be her last chance for

a child – being 46 years old – and because she felt deep down that her baby was really alright. It was a challenge for me because there had been a patient in our service a few years before with a similar diagnosis who did terminate her pregnancy in the second trimester.

The first woman did not terminate her pregnancy as she ultimately came to the place where she felt comfortable, believing that her baby was healthy. She was classified as high risk, by virtue of her age and the sonogram findings. She researched this condition extensively and was well informed. She had several other medical and sonogram evaluations which all agreed with the first. She knew the possibilities, as well as the risks, and her choice in the end was to trust her intuition. Balancing the knowledge afforded by technology with your inner understanding takes courage and clarity. Fortunately, her daughter was born by spontaneous vaginal delivery, without a sign of the identified anomaly, and is now a beautiful, smart 10-year-old.

In the USA, between 14 and 20 weeks' gestation a woman is offered a maternal serum test called an alpha fetoprotein (AFP) or a triple marker test (AFP3) which includes the AFP and levels of two other pregnancy hormones, estriol and human chorionic gonadotrophin (hCG). Some areas are also testing levels of a fourth substance called inhibin-A. High levels of maternal serum AFP can mean the possibility of a neural tube defect (NTD) – this can range from varying degrees of spina bifida to anencephaly, a condition incompatible with life. Other causes of an elevated AFP level are multiple gestation, wrong dates, and some fetal kidney or bowel defects. Abnormally low levels may signify the possibility of Down's syndrome.

Many women find it difficult to understand that this is a screening test, not a diagnostic test. An abnormal result means a possibly increased risk, and strong encouragement to proceed to the next level of testing, which in this case would be a Level 2 sonogram and/or an amniocentesis. (Level 2 sonograms are specifically designed to scan the major organs and markers associated with abnormal AFP levels; amniocentesis is a procedure where amniotic fluid is removed from the uterus through the abdominal wall using a needle and sent for genetic testing.) It also means moving to the next level of explaining risk – very difficult when there is an abnormal result in the picture. At this point an underlying anxiety begins that persists throughout the course of the pregnancy, even if subsequent testing is normal.

When women hear that the test results are abnormal there is an almost universal desire for additional testing to provide reassurance. People interpret information about risk using past experiences, family pressures and their current knowledge. In these instances optimal understanding seems to come from using frequencies rather than probabilities or percentages. Proportions can be confusing, especially with a large denominator. We all experience this in our everyday lives – for example 1/500 sounds and looks like more of a risk than 1/200 because the denominator is larger. In plain English however, 1 in 500 is less of a risk than 1 in 200, and that is understood. To most people 1/25 may sound higher than 4%, because the number 25 is higher than the number 4, even though they are the same.

Generalised information about risk is important to discuss, but personalised risk information is more likely to affect risk reduction behaviour. One-on-one information will also have a stronger effect on the understanding of risk. Several women have confided that despite all the numbers, they feel that for them it is either 100% or 0%. If someone develops a problem or has a baby with a problem, then they can understand this perception – for them it is 100%. It is their baby and their situation. There is no going back. How much control one has over those behaviours and how effective that behaviour will be in reducing the particular risk, are complex interactions that affect the understanding of a risk.

When counselling a woman about an AFP test, it is usual to say that this is an optional test that is offered to pregnant women. The midwife should explain what it is meant to do and what it is not meant to do and what follow-up is available if the result is not normal. She should also point out that a normal test does not

necessarily guarantee a normal baby, nor does an abnormal test mean an abnormal baby.

Women who can read are given written information in their own language if available. After reading the information and reviewing it with the woman, a time for questions is allotted. A significant difficulty is that after the midwife uses the word 'abnormal', anxiety sets in and further communication is blocked. Within this hospital setting if a woman declines the AFP screening test she is asked to sign her name in the chart saying that she has been counselled about the risks and benefits and that her choice is not to have the test. This could seem to be a form of coercion because some women change their minds and say, 'It's just a blood test, right?' The hospital's policy seems to say that if a woman doesn't take this test, the hospital cannot be responsible for any bad outcomes; conversely it also implies that if she does take this test (as is advised) she is guaranteed a healthy baby. Many midwives advise the woman to ask herself what her reaction would be if she had an abnormal outcome, and to consider this before she takes the test.

Once the word 'risk' is spoken, the image of something dangerous and full of peril is present for the remainder of the pregnancy. 'Risk' is characterised as low, medium or high and women usually want to know where they fit in the spectrum. Some women classify themselves in a particular risk category. From personal experience, many women come for their initial visit and say right away, 'I am a high risk pregnancy.' When asked why that is, the variety of answers is astounding, ranging from 'I have anaemia' to one woman who had had three preterm caesarean sections for severe pre-eclampsia/HELLP[5] syndrome, and just about everything in between. Sorting this out takes time because once labelled as 'high risk' it can

---

[5] Pre-eclampsia: previously known as toxaemia; a metabolic disorder characterised by hypertension and proteinuria, can progress rapidly to eclampsia/seizures.
HELLP: Haemolysis, Elevated Liver enzymes, Low Platelet count; a complication of pre-eclampsia involving blood clotting issues.

take until after the normal birth with the normal baby crying in their arms to change that perception of themselves. Whether the label of 'high risk' is given by a physician or a midwife, or taken on by the woman herself because of something she has read or been told, it becomes part of her identity. It seems that some women want to be high risk as the belief is that she will get better care if she is classified as such. As midwives our credibility as valid care providers needs to be established with some women as our birth culture focuses on doctors as the knowledgeable experts, and pregnancy as a medical condition. One midwife colleague I have spoken with feels that even a label of 'low risk' supposes an association of danger because the word 'risk' is based in the language of loss and peril (personal communication, Goodman 2004). This allows fear to hang over the entire process, one that is normal and transformative although certainly not perfect. The woman is just waiting for the moment when something happens and she becomes high risk. To her the use of technology is then justified.

It seems that the language of risk shapes our perceptions of risk, and it is the perception of risk that shapes how we make our choices. Over and over midwife colleagues have told me that risk perception has been moulded by the medicalisation of childbirth. In a routine prenatal visit we may focus on what is going well in the pregnancy as well as what might go wrong, or what is not going right, using parameters such as blood pressure measurement, urine testing, fundal height assessment and weight gain. Midwives will talk a bit about how someone is eating and how to meet the daily requirements for good nutritional status. They review how to assess fetal movement. After this there may not be much time to talk about the emotional changes and social issues that may characterise this pregnancy. Much can be said about what does not happen in a prenatal visit. The time constraints of keeping up patient numbers for optimal clinic operation conflicts with the requirements of many prenatal reimbursement programmes; there is not enough time to do all that is needed. Private practice is not much different,

the expenses of one's own business do not often allow for leisurely discussions.

The arena of malpractice has taken on a personality of its own. It is there, ever present, available to be used in the event of a bad outcome or a less than desired outcome. At times it is a tool used to ease a woman's perception of a looming risk. One example from my own practice was a woman who was demanding that she have a sonogram in the third trimester. She had already had three sonograms showing consistent dating and growth, normal anatomical survey and normal placenta. After it had been explained that it was quite unnecessary (not medically necessary) to have another sonogram, and after all her results had been laid out and reviewed with her, she threatened by saying, 'If there is anything wrong with my baby I'm going to sue you.'

A woman's loss of confidence in her ability to have a normal pregnancy and birth is part of what we are contributing to in our prenatal care design. The risk is inherent in the system, with little effort given to individualising primary care content and most of the focus on development of the regionalised high risk centres. There is that word 'risk' again. We tend to focus on the possibilities of what can go wrong instead of what is going well and how to keep it going well. Midwives are educated to focus on birth as the normal physiological process that it is and to consult and refer for deviations and abnormal findings. Those who are referred are a small group, somewhere between 10% and 20%, and are dependent on definitions which are not completely standardised.

Obstetric training focuses on the pathology of pregnancy and this is what physicians excel at. The education of an obstetrician concentrates on treatment as if the pathology already exists. One noted midwife educator claims:

Obstetrics has intertwined the risk with the pathology as if they were one and the same. They are not. The purpose of the risk assessment was to find predictors of outcomes . . . We used the concept 'predisposing factors' to help us focus on potential problems so we could be ready, just in case . . . But you still treated

the woman as normal until proven otherwise. Now it is just the opposite, all are treated as pathology until proven otherwise . . .
(P. Burkhardt, personal communication 2004)

SOME FINAL THOUGHTS ON RISK

We cannot make our lives risk-free. Although the main purposes of conveying risk information are to allow informed decision-making and to encourage behaviour changes that will limit exposure to adverse events, we cannot completely eliminate risk. The manner in which risk is presented impacts on the interpretation: it is best to use simple explanations in any discussions. The ultimate responsibility in pregnancy and childbirth lies with the parents, however families do look to healthcare providers for guidance. In obstetrics a re-evaluation of risk management and communication strategies would result in a more personalised approach to discussing risk; this would be more likely to influence behaviour change than general population-based risk information.

Ultimately, risk, like beauty is in the eyes of the beholder.
Michael F. Green, MD, Massachusetts General Hospital, Boston, Mass.

References

Adams AM, Smith AF 2001 Risk perception and communication: recent developments and implications for anaesthesia. Anaesthesia 56: 745–755

Bell K, Mill JI 1989 Certified nurse-midwife effectiveness in the HMO Obstetric Team. Obstetrics and Gynecology 74: 112–116

Curzen P et al 1984 Reliability of cardiotocography in predicting baby's condition at birth. British Medical Journal 289: 1345–1347

Dobie SA, Hart LG, Fordyce M et al 1994 Do women choose their obstetric providers based on risks at entry into prenatal care? A study of women in Washington State. Obstetrics and Gynecology 84: 557

Dower CM, Miller JE, O'Neill EH and the Taskforce on Midwifery 1999 Charting a course for the 21st century: the future of midwifery. Pew Health Professions Commission and UCSF Center for the Health Professions, San Francisco

Edwards A, Prior L 1997 Communication about risk-dilemmas for general practitioners. British Journal of General Practice 47: 739–742

Gabay M, Wolfe SM 1995 Encouraging the use of nurse midwives: a report for policy makers. Public Citizens' Health Research Group, Washington, DC

Gabay M, Wolfe SM 1997 Nurse-midwifery, the beneficial alternative. Public Health Reports 112(5): 386–395

Gates EA 2004 Communicating risk in prenatal genetic testing. Journal of Midwifery and Women's Health 49(3): 220–227

Goer H 1995 Obstetric myths vs. research realities – a guide to the medical literature. Bergin & Garvey, Westport, Connecticut

Grant A 1993 Epidemiological principles for the evaluation of monitoring programs – the Dublin experience. Clinical Investigations in Medicine 16(2): 149–158

Greulich B et al 1994 Twelve years and more than 30,000 nurse midwife attended births: the Los Angeles County and USC Women's Hospital Birth Center Experience. Journal of Nurse Midwifery 39: 185–196

Haire D, Elsberry C 1991 Maternity care and outcomes in a high-risk service: the North Central Bronx Experience. Birth 18: 33–37

Law YY, Lam KY 1999 A randomized controlled trial comparing midwife-managed care and obstetrician-managed care for women assessed to be at low risk in the initial intrapartum period. Journal of Obstetric and Gynecology Research 25(2): 107–112

MacDorman MF, Singh GK 1998 Midwifery care, social and medical risk factors, and birth outcomes in the United States. Journal of Epidemiology and Community Health 52(5): 310–323

National Center for Health Statistics, Centers for Disease Control and Prevention 2005 Live births by place of delivery, and attendant, according to race and Hispanic origin (Tables 1–24). Online. Available: www.cdc.gov/nchs/data/statab/t001x24.pdf

Oakley D, Murray ME, Murtland T et al 1996 Comparisons of outcomes of maternity care by obstetricians and certified nurse-midwives. Obstetrics and Gynecology 88(5): 823–829

Rooks JP 1997 Midwifery and childbirth in America. Temple University Press, Philadelphia

Rosen MG, Dickinson JC 1993 The paradox of EFM: more data may not enable us to predict or prevent infant neurologic morbidity. American Journal of Obstetrics and Gynecology 168(3 pt 1): 745–751

Rosen MG, Hobel CJ 1986 Prenatal and perinatal factors associated with brain disorders. Obstetrics and Gynecology 68(3): 416–421

Rothman BK 1991 In labor – women and power in the birthplace. WW Norton, New York

Sandmire HF 1990 Whither electronic fetal monitoring? Obstetrics and Gynecology 76(6): 1130–1134

Schlenzka PF 1999 Safety of alternative approaches to childbirth. Stanford University Press, Palo Alto, California. Summary online. Available: http://www.vbfree.org/docs/schlenzka.htm

Speert H 1980 Midwives, nurses and nurse-midwives 1980 Obstetrics & gynecology in America: a history. ACOG, Chicago

State of Washington Department of Licensing 1988 An assessment of childbirth outcomes in Washington. Report to the Legislature SSB 5163, State of Washington, USA

Strong TH, Jr 2000 Expecting trouble, what expectant parents should know about prenatal care in America. NYU Press, New York, NY, USA, p 1

Sykes GS et al 1983 Fetal distress and the condition of newborn infants. British Medical Journal 287: 943–945

Thacker SB 1987 The efficacy of intrapartum EFM. American Journal of Obstetrics and Gynecology 156(1): 24–30

US Senate Congressional Hearings 1978 Obstetrical practices in the United States, a hearing before the Subcommittee on Health and Scientific Research of the Committee on Human Resources. 95th Congress, US Senate, 17 Apr

Van Tuinen I, Wolfe SM 1992 Unnecessary cesarean sections: halting a national epidemic. Public Citizen's Health Research Group, Washington DC

Wagner M 1994 Pursuing the birth machine, the search for appropriate birth technology, ACE Graphics, Australia

Further Reading

Aalfs CM, Mollema ED et al 2004 Genetic counseling for familial conditions during pregnancy: an analysis of patient characteristics. Clinical Genetics 66: 112–121

Jeffcott M 2002 Examining the role of risk perception in the use of obstetric technology. WWDU International Conference, University of Glasgow, p 3

McCormack M (ed) 2000 Managing complications in pregnancy and childbirth: a guide for midwives and doctors. World Health Organization, Geneva

Ocean J 2004 Change, risk, trust. La Trobe University, Auckland

Redman C, Walker I 1992 Pre eclampsia – the facts. Oxford University Press, Oxford

Rothman BK 1999 Recreating motherhood: ideology and technology in a patriarchal society. Norton, New York

Spurgeon P, Hicks C, Barwell F 2001 Antenatal delivery and postnatal comparisons of maternal satisfaction with two pilot Changing Childbirth schemes compared with a traditional model of care. Midwifery 17(2): 123–132

Turnbull D, Holmes A, Shields N et al 1996 Randomized, controlled trial of efficacy of midwife-managed care. Lancet 348(9022): 213–218

Chapter **14**

Risk and Choice: Knowledge and Control

Andrew Symon

INTRODUCTION

The chapters in this book have examined the concepts of risk and choice from a number of perspectives. We have seen how the language of risk and choice in relation to maternity care has been used in several countries. We have heard the voice of midwives, obstetricians, those engaged in risk management, and those who advocate on behalf of pregnant women and new mothers. Throughout all these different accounts, stories and explanations, there are two essential themes: knowledge, and control (sometimes referred to as power). These two features can be said to be symbiotically linked, each one feeding into the other. From the point of view of deciding where we are in the risk/choice debate, it is useful to clarify who has the knowledge and who has the control. It is also pertinent to ask how these are expressed.

We have seen that there are many 'takes' on the question of how risk and choice are balanced. The doctrine of risk has been rather easier to explore than the matter of choice, especially from the point of view of healthcare practitioners, and this in itself tells a story. The evolution of risk management, and in particular clinical risk management, has been significantly affected by the health service's experience (or perception) of litigation. Referring to the UK, Walshe & Sheldon (1998: 18) claim that 'it has been largely the financial pressure from legal actions for clinical negligence which has driven the NHS to take risk and risk management seriously.' Certainly the picture within maternity care in Britain changed significantly in the 1990s, and there was an awareness (sometimes used as a backdrop to the discussion about litigation) that practitioners were more conscious of the concept of risk. This was summed up memorably by one midwife whom I interviewed in exploratory research in the early 1990s (Symon 1994). She told me: 'We don't take risks so much now – although risk isn't quite the right word.' Her unwillingness to acknowledge that risk was 'the right word' illustrated the unease of the whole subject, and is reflected in Bastian's (2003) comment that people are afraid to take risks. Practitioners were aware that the way in which they practised, and the way this appeared to others, were both crucial, but along with this awareness there was an edgy defensiveness.

THE RISE OF RISK MANAGEMENT

The first half of the 1990s in Britain saw a great deal of debate about how maternity services should be organised and delivered, a debate which culminated in the declaration that 'the three Cs' (choice, continuity and control) were paramount considerations. However, since that time 'risk' seems to have made its mark on the consciousness of practitioners more emphatically than 'choice'. As noted in the first chapter of this book, there are books and journals dedicated to risk and risk management; there are also websites (the term 'clinical risk management' in an internet search engine produced over 90 000 hits) discussing general and specific perinatal risk issues. The language of risk has become adopted almost wholesale, and few if any practitioners will be unaware of the existence and role of the clinical risk manager. Ranged against this is the argument advancing the cause of choice, whose principal weapon until the recent appearance of Mavis Kirkham's *Informed Choice in Maternity Care* may well have been the admirable *Informed Choice* leaflets produced by MIDIRS. Sad to report, it has been difficult to prove any significant benefit from

these leaflets, despite their comprehensive nature (O'Cathain et al 2002, Wiggins & Newburn 2004). This experience suggests that risk is a more powerful driver for health service providers than the consideration of choice. This may be because service providers have been heavily influenced by the developing clinical risk management industry; being involved in the service for many years on end (while user involvement is necessarily more short-term), means that the impact of this approach becomes embedded and is therefore more powerful than the stance of service users.

Whether the implementation of risk management as a response to the perceived increase in litigation was effective in reducing claims or the amount paid out in compensation is disputed by Tingle (2003: 18):

> It is interesting to note that there is a clinical negligence crisis in the US, despite the fact that they have had a much longer time to develop health risk management strategies than we have had in the UK.

Additionally, Merritt et al (1999) note that while clinical practice guidelines and care pathways had been introduced to improve quality of care, reduce healthcare costs, and limit malpractice liability, there was minimal evidence to support the contention that outcomes (in their study neonatal ones) had benefited from their implementation.

Whether litigation was the most significant driver behind the development of risk management, or whether the inevitable expansion of a large 'risk bureaucracy' merely used this as a fig leaf, it is worth considering some of the features of this phenomenon. For the person or family pursuing a claim, the trauma is multifaceted: an injury (usually physical) causing long-term anguish, and protracted emotional trauma are the minimum; financial hardship may also be experienced. There is loss of confidence in a system which is said to be there to help but which, when the legal battle lines are drawn, can appear obstructive and unhelpful (Symon 2001). From the health service's point of view, legal claims against practitioners carry a great deal of baggage: there is the trauma of possible guilt or damaged reputations for individuals; the undoubted expense (particularly severe in perinatal claims); and the loss of corporate reputation, as individual units are associated with poor outcomes and legal argument. There are really few winners in such scenarios, although the lawyers often get accused of this.

THE SYSTEM

The reaction from the health service's perspective was to attempt to minimise the likelihood of such occurrences – in itself an entirely laudable aim. In this book, Kennedy (Chapter 2) has explained that the conceptual basis on which risk management rests is 'the system'. Risk management, he says, is a response to uncertainty, 'and can be considered to be an attempt to impose order'. This is not problematic in many situations: for example, we want the train driver or airline pilot to know about certain risks and trust him/her to take steps to manage these so that we arrive safely at our destination. Where it can become a problem is in the way 'the system' tends to claim for itself the highest levels of knowledge on which decisions about imposing order or about clinical care are made. An uneasy feeling can also accompany this attempt to control uncertainty: are choices only offered when 'the system' thinks it can control or predict or otherwise be certain of the outcome? O'Boyle (Chapter 3) referred to the view that practitioners may only provide those options that are convenient to them. One could substitute the word 'practical' for 'convenient': Cameron and Ellwood have shown how weather conditions can affect the availability of services in remote and rural areas; Smith has also noted that a system with limited resources may arrive at the stage where options do become restricted. This has been seen in reports of health authorities 'refusing' to allow women a home birth because of lack of staff (AIMS 2000).

There is an uncomfortable juxtaposition in the idea of 'the system' organising things when trying to guarantee individualised care, and this is not because the goals are different. Various players involved in healthcare come at it from all sorts of angles, but all with the best of motives: in maternity care this would normally be expressed as wanting to have a live and healthy mother and baby, and for the mother the memory of a good experience. That is hardly controversial, and yet throughout this book we have seen how different viewpoints about how best to achieve this have at times led to tension and pain. The root of this tension would appear to be the competing claims concerning the validity of different forms of knowledge. This was well demonstrated in Chapter 4 by Edwards and Murphy-Lawless, where women's stories about claiming knowledge about birth clashed with systems approaches that are designed to maximise good clinical outcomes on a population level. Adams (2003: 5) talks of the 'hierarchist' view of risk management, where it is the job of those in authority to consider risk management issues because 'the ignorant lay public cannot be relied upon to interpret the evidence correctly or use it responsibly.' However well-intentioned the design, there is ample evidence from several countries that 'the system' can generate its own problems which actually make poor outcomes more likely, as root cause analysis has demonstrated (Reason 2001). This is in fact particularly likely in complex multidisciplinary areas such as maternity care when clinical emergencies arise.

As I noted in the introductory chapter, practitioners are inducted into a system based largely on epidemiological knowledge. There is also the paradox that most clinical education (for doctors at least) occurs at the acute care level, whereas in pregnancy most of the clinical care does not take place in the acute hospital setting. This can result in very differing viewpoints about normality, autonomy and control. The system attempts to achieve outcomes based on utilitarian grounds – the best possible outcome for the greatest number – and on one level that argument is difficult to dismiss. If we want to tackle significant problems, we begin by trying to maximise good outcomes for as many people as possible. In crisis situations there is little doubt about what this means – as many lives as possible must be saved as expeditiously as is practicable. It is salutary to be reminded of the devastating maternal health statistics in parts of sub-Saharan Africa, for example. Having worked in that part of the world it is impossible not to be conscious of the overwhelming problems encountered by so many. We are indeed fortunate to be considering questions of risk and choice from a comparatively safe standpoint, where maternal death during childbirth is extremely rare, and where there is a reasonable expectation that a baby born at term will survive and flourish.

From this perspective, it is easy to see that the intended goals of service users and providers are not oppositional. There is, nevertheless, some room for dissension over the best means of achieving the desired clinical outcome.

POLITICAL OR PERSONAL?

To return to the question of who decides the best route, some insight into the matter of hierarchical knowledge can be gleaned from Agustsson's assertion (Chapter 9) that where safe options are available, women should be empowered to express their preferences. The question is then raised: who decides what constitutes safety? To take one example, how are decisions about mode of birth to be decided when it is suspected that a fetus is large? A midwife or obstetrician might, on the basis of ultrasound and other clinical evidence, believe that the best way of avoiding shoulder dystocia and the possibility of a baby with Erb's palsy, and a mother with significant perineal trauma, is to plan for an elective caesarean. Nobody would question the desire to minimise the occurrence of these traumatic clinical outcomes, but there may be several other unintended consequences in terms of morbidity arising from the caesarean itself. This is quite apart from the implicit assumption that the knowledge underpinning the practitioner's view is a superior form of knowledge to that of the woman who may decide that she is capable of a safe vaginal birth.

Kennedy reminds us in Chapter 2 that, from a risk management perspective, 'risk is a

political concept, and failures are therefore fundamentally political events.' However, risk can also be considered a personal concept. 'The system' tries to define, conceptualise and manage something, but it sees things in terms of aggregates, not in individual terms. Could industrial-sized healthcare systems, based as they are on serving large populations, do anything else? Pilley Edwards and Murphy-Lawless (Chapter 4) tell us that risk protocols and evidence-based care (the greatest claim to superior knowledge) are too often incompatible with choice, especially if women make decisions that fall outside these protocols and evidence. Walsh (2003: 474) has noted elsewhere that:

> Risk management needs to be exposed as not objective, rational and value-free, but as socially constructed, biased to certain values and politically motivated to reinforce the powerful in health care.

McNally's (Chapter 6) assertion that women in her unit are not given any choice as to whether cord blood gas analysis is performed reveals the continued existence of a cautious and paternalistic approach to risk management.

Does it all then boil down to Quilliam's (1999: 282) simple – but not simplistic – question: 'Will it happen to me?' The cautious optimism of the mother espousing 'birth wisdom' can be contrasted with the more pessimistic stance of the practitioner as she monitors the labour of what Walsh has, in this book, called the 'not yet ill patient'. The belief that it will or will not happen may be a very powerful driver, and this belief, or even knowledge, may dictate what the woman will consent to, and indeed how much control she asserts over events. The same belief may determine what a practitioner does, and certainly the rise in defensive clinical practices within maternity care was evident by the 1990s (Symon 2000, 2001).

There are many possible difficulties with imposing order based on supposedly superior knowledge. Clinical guidelines, arising as they do from the best available research evidence, must still acknowledge that research knowledge is always partial, and its conclusions or recommendations may not apply in every case.

Cameron and Ellwood (Chapters 11 and 12) have recounted how these debates may be seen from different angles – there are statistical data and personal data. For some indigenous Australians the belief that it is spiritually and culturally important to birth 'on country' may override 'scientific' calculations about risk factors. It may well be posited that Western knowledge has tried to isolate physical health outcomes as the predominant feature, and accordingly downplays the significance of emotional or spiritual wellbeing. While a holistic approach disputes this, there is little doubt that clinical guidelines give greatest prominence to physical parameters. Pilley Edwards and Murphy-Lawless (Chapter 4) claim that women are asking for a reconnection of birth physiology with the emotional needs of women, noting that such skills and 'birth wisdom' have largely disappeared. Practitioners may espouse the knowledge of scientific findings, while some women at least express the optimism of 'birth wisdom' – believing that childbirth will usually turn out well, but one is prepared just in case ('watchful waiting'). How then do the various parties in this debate attempt to communicate with each other?

MAKING CONNECTIONS

Communication between practitioners and pregnant women has not always been constructive and effective. Viisainen's (2000: 810) reference to practitioner criticisms of parents' 'non-compliant behaviour' has been alluded to by Pilley Edwards and Murphy-Lawless (Chapter 4). My own early research in this area, conducted in 1991, involved interviewing midwives and obstetricians. One midwife commented:

Sometimes I feel the women are – God forgive me – very very selfish; I think they're all into the way they want it.

Others said:

I also blame the media . . . for misconceptions about pregnancy and childbirth; they give a very – and I have to use the word – ignorant

viewpoint. . . . I think (this) is creating a very false impression, and we deal with it every day in here . . . They would like it to be all natural, no pain, no need for analgesia: the baby just comes out and that's it. It's not a realistic picture at all . . .

The clients we have are much more informed . . . they have more ideas of what they want, and they become very dissatisfied when it doesn't work out the way they want it to.

Here we get a lot of 'elderly primigravida', where they're 37, 40. They've got great careers, and they've got their own lives sorted out, and they come in here and they have great expectations – abnormal expectations – and it falls flat on them . . .

(Symon 1992, 1994)

These quotes paint a picture of demanding but ill-informed women who assert their rights regardless of the likely clinical consequences, and there seems little doubt that some practitioners took some time to acknowledge the shifting power base within maternity care. I should stress that these interviews took place some time ago, and I would hope that current views are more understanding of different viewpoints. It may have been that midwives in the early 1990s had little experience of women opting for anything other than the set menu. However, even today, as Pilley Edwards and Murphy-Lawless (Chapter 4) and O'Connor (Chapter 10) note, women who wish to have their babies outside a conventional hospital setting, or who opt for an alternative to unit protocols, are still seen by some as awkward.

This comes down to the knowledge on which such wishes are based, and how it is expressed. Some may assert that there is a reclaiming of the 'birth wisdom' that was ousted by the growth of technocratic childbirth, itself heralded in Britain by the 1970s move to reduce or even eliminate home birth. But on what is that 'birth wisdom' based? Is there an innate sense of potential accomplishment, albeit one that was all but eradicated by the advent of 'managed' birth? As noted above in the context of Australia, Cameron and Ellwood (Chapters 11 and 12) have indicated an indigenous cultural take on the most appropriate approach to childbirth. There may clearly be specific issues that are particular to certain groups. Cameron and Ellwood have also told us that there is no such concept as percentage in the language of indigenous Australians, and so the use of percentages is meaningless in trying to convey the concept of risk. Indeed, in a multicultural society, it can be very difficult to present an understanding of risk which will be appreciated by all, something Brooks (Chapter 13) alluded to in her discussion of trying to convey clinical risk factors to women from ethnic minorities who define 'risk' (good or bad) in the context of their home traditions, which may reflect very different healthcare systems. In fact, as Brooks has reported, and as I noted in the introductory chapter, the very word 'risk' may be part of the problem, as it has negative connotations. Language can convey unintended meanings which themselves reinforce the power differential in clinical care. Women may be put on trial (e.g. trial of labour, trial of scar), with the parameters of judgment being determined by practitioners. Women may be deemed to fail (e.g. failed induction, failure to progress), language which can, however unintentionally, demean.

The pregnant woman and the practitioner may have imperfect understanding when they speak different languages (and Brooks noted how difficult it can be to convey nuances of risk in another tongue (Chapter 13)), but there may also be mis-communication even when they speak the same language. Smith's fictitious (but reality-based) scenario of a woman living on an island and wanting a home birth despite the potential difficulties in travelling to the nearest obstetric unit, illustrated how considerable effort may be required to arrive at a mutually acceptable arrangement. In her scenario the midwife was flexible, negotiating and facilitating – surely a model for effective care. To do this she needed to know what was desirable and what was practicable. Sharing this knowledge effectively with both the woman and the hospital was essential. In this vein, Kirkham & Stapleton (2004) report that midwives often find themselves in this negotiator's 'middle ground'.

This exemplary situation, where the woman is fully aware and therefore in a position to make an informed decision, contrasts with the example given by Rich (Chapter 5), where, in the best tradition of paternalistic medicine, a doctor claimed that at times 'It's better you don't know'. He also notes that the timing of information giving is critical, and that practitioners should not assume that just because they have told the woman something she has understood and will remember this.

Rich claims that women can be helped to make realistic choices only when they have full knowledge of possible complications. The guarding of knowledge by practitioners (thereby perhaps retaining a sense of control) sits uneasily with the contemporary tendency to make information available, although the tone of the information giving (whether intentional or unintentional) can be significant. The Royal College of Midwives has noted that 'women tend towards compliance if they are led to believe that they or especially their baby is at risk' (RCM 2000: 8). The RCM acknowledges that midwifery care should be 'centred on each woman's unique and individual needs' (RCM 2002), suggesting that women must be listened to and their views accorded respect. Similarly, a recent Clinical Governance Advice paper from the Royal College of Obstetricians and Gynaecologists (2005: 3) notes that 'A safety culture is more likely to flourish where there is strong leadership, teamwork, communication, user involvement and training.' How much user involvement there is, and what form this takes, is debatable, but this is essential if connections are to be made.

Rich points out that service users need information in order to make choices, but that choices can be limited. Much of the debate about choice centres on what women deemed to be 'low risk' might want or ought to be able to achieve. What happens then when circumstances restrict this? There is a conundrum in that many women are choosing to leave pregnancies until later in life, but this in itself reduces their scope for choice when they do become pregnant, because they are statistically more at risk of complications. He notes that some women, having experienced problems during pregnancy, are choosing not to have a subsequent pregnancy. The exercise of choice, then, can be about avoiding a problem, not opting for something desirable.

CONCLUSION

It is tempting to conclude that the focus on risk management, albeit unwittingly, has led to a situation where the imperative is always to control rather than to facilitate birth; to a situation where women's 'knowledge' about what they can achieve in childbirth is discounted in favour of a purportedly 'objective' knowledge designed to achieve population-based outcomes. The individual woman's knowledge may not guarantee the desired outcome (sometimes the charge levelled against 'allowing' women to decide the venue of birth, for example), but then neither does the supposedly superior objective knowledge of clinical expertise, with all its technological gadgetry. Babies die and suffer handicaps even when the whole panoply of obstetric, anaesthetic or paediatric interventions is available.

When there are acknowledged problems there is rarely any real disagreement about the appropriate course of action: there's no one who wouldn't want a well-oiled machine to be working when the emergency happens. In such a situation we want an expert to be in charge – which means being in control. In this circumstance of 'necessity' (and this was covered by O'Boyle in Chapter 3) there really are no dissenters: we are grateful for the life-saving expertise that is available.

The debate is really about where the bar is in relation to such problems; about whether the individual woman intuitively or objectively knows more about her situation and what is right for her than the cover-all policies of a maternity unit. This is where the doctrine of 'tools, not rules' applies: protocols and guidelines are not supposed to be used as blunt instruments, although the reality of 'regulatory creep' suggests that what may start out as signposts and guidance can turn into more dogmatic instructions.

However, throughout this book there has been ample evidence that the individual approach that is theoretically on offer in maternity care is not guaranteed; that claims to knowledge by pregnant women and practitioners are not always evenly considered; and that choice has had less impact on the delivery of maternity care than considerations of risk. Indeed, risk management is such a powerful driver within healthcare that it may be said that risk is the tail that wags the healthcare dog.

References

Adams J 2003 In defence of bad luck. Online. Available: www.spiked-online.com 8 Dec 2005

AIMS (Association for Improvements in the Maternity Services) 2000 A nail in the coffin for home birth. AIMS Journal 12(3). Online. Available: http://www.aims.org.uk/Journal/Vol12No3/ukcc.htm

Bastian H 2003 Variation in perceptions of risk between doctors and patients: risks look different when they are close to home. Australian Prescriber 26(1): 20–21

Kirkham M, Stapleton H 2004 The culture of maternity services in Wales and England as a barrier to informed choice. In: Kirkham M (ed) Informed choice in maternity care. Palgrave Macmillan, Basingstoke

Merritt TA, Gold M, Holland J 1999 A critical evaluation of clinical practice guidelines in neonatal medicine: does their use improve quality and lower costs? Journal of Evaluation in Clinical Practice 5(2): 169–177

MIDIRS Informed choice. Online. Available: http://www.midirs.org/

O'Cathain A, Walters SJ, Nicholl JP et al 2002 Use of evidence based leaflets to promote informed choice in maternity care: randomised controlled trial in everyday practice. British Medical Journal 324: 643

Quilliam S 1999 Clinical risk management in midwifery: what are midwives for? MIDIRS Midwifery Digest 9: 280–284

RCM (Royal College of Midwives) 2000 Reassessing risk: a midwifery perspective. RCM, London

RCM 2002 Refocusing the role of the midwife (Position Paper 26). RCM, London

RCOG (Royal College of Obstetricians and Gynaecologists) 2005 Improving patient safety: risk management for maternity and gynaecology

(Clinical Governance Advice No 2, Oct). RCOG, London

Reason J 2001 Understanding adverse events: the human factor. In: Vincent C (ed) Clinical risk management: enhancing patient safety. BMJ Books, London, p 9–30

Symon A 1992 Who's accountable? Who's to blame? MA (Hons) dissertation, University of Edinburgh (unpublished)

Symon A 1994 Midwives and litigation 2: a small-scale survey of attitudes. British Journal of Midwifery 2(4): 176–181

Symon A 2000 Litigation and defensive clinical practice: quantifying the problem. Midwifery 16: 8–14

Symon A 2001 Obstetric litigation from A-Z. Salisbury, Quay Books

Tingle J 2003 Is risk management really working? Health Care Risk Report 9(3): 18

Viisainen K 2000 The moral dangers of home birth: parents' perceptions of risks in home birth in Finland. Sociology of Health and Illness 22(6): 792–814

Walsh D 2003 Risk management is not objective (editorial). British Journal of Midwifery 11(8): 474

Walshe K, Sheldon T 1998 Dealing with clinical risk: implications of the rise of evidence-based health care. Public Money and Management Oct–Dec: 15–20

Wiggins M, Newburn M 2004 Information used by pregnant women, and their understanding and use of evidence-based Informed Choice leaflets. In: Kirkham M (ed) Informed choice in maternity care. Palgrave Macmillan, Basingstoke

Index